The Mind Object

The Mind Object

Precocity and Pathology of Self-Sufficiency

edited by
Edward G. Corrigan, Ph.D.
Pearl-Ellen Gordon, Ph.D.

JASON ARONSON INC.
Northvale, New Jersey
London

The editors gratefully acknowledge permission to reprint excerpts from "Interior" by Dorothy Parker, from *The Portable Dorothy Parker* by Dorothy Parker, introduction by Brendan Gill. Copyright © 1928, renewed © 1956 by Dorothy Parker. Used by permission of Viking Penguin, a division of Penguin Books USA Inc., and Gerald Duckworth & Co. Ltd., London, UK.

This book was set in 11 pt. Bodoni Antiqua by Alpha Graphics of Pittsfield, New Hampshire, and printed and bound by Book-mart Press of North Bergen, New Jersey.

Library of Congress Cataloging-in-Publication Data

The mind object : precocity and pathology of self-sufficiency / edited by Edward G. Corrigan and Pearl-Ellen Gordon.
    p. cm.
    Includes bibliographical references and index.
    ISBN 1-56821-480-4 (alk. paper)
    1. Object relations (Psychoanalysis)   2. Ego (Psychology)
3. Object constancy (Psychoanalysis)   I. Corrigan, Edward G.
II. Gordon, Pearl-Ellen.
BF175.5.O24M56   1995
150.19'5—dc20   95-9997

Manufactured in the United States of America. Jason Aronson Inc. offers books and cassettes. For information and catalog write to Jason Aronson Inc., 230 Livingston Street, Northvale, New Jersey 07647.

CONTENTS

ACKNOWLEDGMENTS

There are many friends and colleagues whose encouragement and support we wish to acknowledge, but especially the authors who have taken up this subject and offered their original papers. Christopher Bollas saw in our work on the "mind object" the possibility of a book and with his characteristic generosity, humor, and intelligence he has seen us through this project. Adam Phillips always refers to this book as "our book," and we share that sentiment with him, thanking him for his spirited backing. Harold Boris, who joined this project after many of the papers were written, read and referred to several of them in his own paper. We want to acknowledge his special effort; his contribution works as a broad discussion of the book while remaining a distinctly Harold Boris essay.

In our roles as officers of the Section for Childhood and Adolescence, the Division of Psychoanalysis, the American Psychological Association, and in involvement with scientific programs for the Society of the Institute for Contemporary Psychotherapy, we had the opportunity of meeting many of the contributors to this volume. Through our participation in the Section for Childhood and Adolescence we developed the idea of a national study group for members of the section. In our initial planning, our colleague and friend Carol Kaye suggested that we study precocious ego development, a clinically familiar but unexamined phenomenon. We met as a national study group on a regular basis at the Spring meetings of Division 39, beginning in Boston in 1989. Christopher Bollas was a consultant at this first meeting. Although many colleagues joined us at our national meetings, our core study group was made up of Peter Shabad and Stanley Selinger in Chicago, Ira Schaer in Detroit, Stephen Seligman in San Francisco, and Carol Kaye, Ruth Rosenthal, Richard Eichler, and Donna Bassin along with ourselves in New York. Eventually, we presented our findings in formal presentations at the Spring Meetings in Chicago in 1991 and Philadelphia in 1992.

We would like to thank our colleagues with whom we have discussed the case of Simon: Anni Bergman, Christopher Bollas, Susan Coates, Peter Neubauer, Margaret Rustin, Martin Silverman, Sabrina Wolf, and Larry Zelnick, as well as the members of our monthly child discussion group, David Beyda, Elsa First, Carol Kaye, and David Pollens.

Finally, we wish to express our gratitude to Michael Moskowitz at Jason Aronson and Cesare Sacerdoti at Karnac Books for their immediate and enthusiastic support.

CONTRIBUTORS

Christopher Bollas is a member of the British Psycho-Analytical Society and author of *The Shadow of the Object, Forces of Destiny, Being a Character, Cracking Up* and co-author with David Sundelson of *The New Informants*.

Harold N. Boris is a member of the psychology faculty in the Department of Psychiatry of the Harvard Medical School at the Cambridge Hospital and author of *Passions of the Mind, Sleights of Mind*, and *Envy*.

Nina Coltart was a psychoanalyst for thirty-five years before her recent retirement. She was a training analyst at the British Psycho-Analytical Society where she was also Chair of the Board and Council and Vice President. Dr. Coltart was Director of the London Clinic of Psycho-Analysis for ten years. She is author of *Slouching Towards Bethlehem* and *How to Survive as a Psychotherapist* and is working on a third book.

Edward Corrigan is supervisor and faculty member at the Institute for Contemporary Psychotherapy in New York City and faculty member at the National Institutes for Psychoanalysis and former President of the Section for Childhood and Adolescence, Division of Psychoanalysis, of the American Psychological Association.

Michael Eigen is a control and training analyst at the National Psychological Association for Psychoanalysis and Associate Clinical Professor, New York University Postdoctoral Program in Psychoanalysis and Psychotherapy. He is author of *The Psychotic Core, Coming Through the Whirlwind*, and *The Electrified Tightrope*.

Pearl-Ellen Gordon is a member of the Executive Committee, Director of Child and Adolescent Treatment, faculty member, and supervisor at The Institute for Contemporary Psychotherapy in New York City. She is also currently President of the Section for Childhood and Adolescence, Division of Psychoanalysis, of the American Psychological Association.

Adam Phillips is Principal Child Psychotherapist in the Wolverton Gardens Child and Family Consultation Centre. He is author of *Winnicott, On Kissing, Tickling and Being Bored, On Flirtation,* and forthcoming, *Terrors and Experts.*

Ira Schaer is a member of the staff and faculty, Children's Service, Detroit Psychiatric Institute, and President-Elect of the Section for Childhood and Adolescence, Division of Psychoanalysis, of the American Psychological Association.

Stephen Seligman is Clinical Professor of Psychiatry at the Infant–Parent Program, San Francisco General Hospital, University of California, Faculty member of the Psychoanalytic Institute of Northern California, and Associate Member of the San Francisco Psychoanalytic Institute.

Stanley Selinger is Clinical Assistant Professor of Psychology at the University of Illinois at Chicago and Section Head of Psychology at Christ Hospital in Oak Lawn, Illinois. He is past president of the Chicago Association for Psychoanalytic Psychology.

Peter Shabad is senior staff psychologist, child and adolescent inpatient psychiatry of the Michael Reese Hospital and Medical School, and Assistant Professor in the Department of Psychiatry at Northwestern University Medical School. He is co-editor of *The Problems of Loss and Mourning* and author of *The Echo of Inner Truth* (forthcoming).

Harold Stewart is a training analyst of the British Psycho-Analytical Society and Chairman of its Education Committee. He was, until his recent retirement, Consultant Psychotherapist at the Tavistock

Clinic. He is author of *Psychic Experience and Problems of Technique* and *From Primary Love to the Basic Fault: The Work of Michael Balint* (forthcoming).

Maria St. John is an Infant Development Specialist, Children's Hospital, Oakland, California; infant–parent psychotherapy trainee, Infant–Parent Program, San Francisco General Hospital, University of California, San Francisco.

Raymond Vasser is a Ph.D candidate in clinical psychology, University of Detroit-Mercy and clinical psychologist, William Beaumont Hospital, Royal Oak, Michigan.

INTRODUCTION

Her mind lives tidily, apart
From cold and noise and pain,
And bolts the door against her heart,
Out wailing in the rain.
            —D. Parker, "Interior"

Anthony, a young adult in the third year of analysis, is discussing his tendencies toward addictive behaviors and their impact on his body when he suddenly realizes, as he put it, that "my body is not part of me—it is a thing that I have." Toward the end of the session he comments, "I am always more connected to my mind than my body. . . . I have totally blocked my body as part of me. . . . I exist through my mind." He underscores this point in the next session when he ends a long silence by remarking that he will "never progress through silence." All he hears is his mind questioning him: "What are you doing? . . . You will never get anywhere this way, dummy!"

Can a person relate to his mind as an object—depend upon it to the exclusion of other objects—idealize it, fear it, hate it? Can a person live out a life striving to attain the elusive power of his mind's perfection, yielding to its promise while sacrificing the body's truth?

We have asked a distinguished group of clinicians, whose work is located within the object relations tradition, to explore these questions within the domain of their own clinical experience. The resulting essays reflect the individuality and creativity of the authors, as they examine, clinically and theoretically, the concept of the mind as an object.

Winnicott (1949), in his seminal paper, "Mind and Its Relation to the Psyche-Soma," was the first to describe how very early in life an individual can, in response to environmental failure, turn away from the body and its needs and establish "mental functioning as a thing in itself." Winnicott's elusive term, the *mind psyche*, describes a subtle, yet fundamentally violent split in which the mind negates the role of the body, its feelings, and functions as the source of creative living. "The mind in such a case has a false function and a life of its own, and it dominates the psyche-soma instead of being a special function of the psyche-soma" (Winnicott 1988, p. 140). Elaborating upon Winnicott's notions of precocious mental functioning, Masud Khan (1971) speaks of a "precocious structuralization of the developmental process," a "rigid premature structuring of internalized primary objects and fantasies and a negativity toward all new experience and object-relations" (p. 220).

We feel the time has come to extend Winnicott and Khan's ideas and introduce the concept of the mind object. We have chosen this clinically meaningful term not only to signify the central dissociation, the mind separated from the body, but also to underscore its function. As Adam Phillips explains (Chapter 11) "In 'health,' one might say using Winnicott's medical language, the mind listens to and collaborates with the body and its objects (or rather, subjects); in 'illness' there is a military coup and a dictator is installed called a mind-object, at once bureaucrat and terrorist."

When the mind "takes on a life of its own," it becomes an object —separate, as it were, from the self. And because it is an object that originates as a substitute for maternal care, it becomes an object of intense attachment—turned to for security, solace, and gratification. Significantly, having achieved the status of an object, the mind can also turn on the self—attacking, demeaning, and persecuting the individual. And once this object relationship is established, it organizes the self, providing an aura of omnipotence; but this precocious, schizoid solution is basically an illusion, vulnerable to breakdown and the anxieties associated with breakdown. In Chapter 1, we review in greater detail the literature on precocious development and discuss central anxieties and defenses as well as treatment dilemmas that we have encountered in child and adult patients who have turned to their mind as an object.

The cast of adult characters who are introduced in this book presents us with new and clinically useful ways of viewing the schizoid, depressive, narcissistic, and obsessive-compulsive patient in terms of the self's relationship to the mind. Harold Stewart (Chapter 3) discusses a period in the analysis of a female patient in the process of relinquishing the "superiority" of her mind. She is in a regressed state of uncertainty and paranoid suspiciousness and thrown back into the confused childhood states against which the mind object had defended. Nina Coltart (Chapter 2) and Harold Boris (Chapter 9) detail their long and painstaking work with brilliant obsessive-compulsive men, the philosopher and the teacher, highlighting with precision the mind object at work. By idealizing their minds, each became, in Boris's words, "a prisoner of his sanctuary."

Christopher Bollas (Chapter 5) places us in the internal world of Helmut, the tortured depressive, whose mind is at war with the self, berating, belittling, rendering him helplessly immobilized. Michael Eigen's (Chapter 6) female patient, ever distrustful of the intellect and its destructive potential, has turned to a life of intense feeling and looks initially very different from the patients described by the other authors. Nevertheless, her treatment unmasked a "hidden omniscience and tyrannical sense of rightness parasitically embedded in mystical feeling." Unearthed was a secret mind object, moralistic and judgmental.

The three child cases that are presented (Chapters 4, 7, and 8) Simon, Tony, and Dorian, permit us to view the early organization of the mind object. Through imitation, omnipotent fantasy, and acts of self-sufficiency, Simon attempts to obliterate his mother and substitute his mind as his most important object—at one moment, an adored, magical protector, at another, an abusive attacker. Schaer and Vasser describe Tony, a streetwise 7-year-old from the inner city, charming, manipulative, masterful at concealing any vulnerability, who amazingly looks and acts like a much older boy. We are struck by the power of his mind to thwart and negate the child in the child, as he has literally, in mind and body, grown up too fast. Seligman and St. John present a session with the superficially plucky and congenial toddler Dorian. We can see in her frantic and hyperenergized play, through which she takes over the role of the other, the foreclosure of authentic self-experience. There is no baby.

In the clinical chapters the authors elucidate many technical issues that arise in work with these patients as they confront the power of the intellect to stimulate and seduce, on the one hand, and, on the other, to deaden and destroy. The complex counter-transference feelings that are stirred by these patients are movingly portrayed. Coltart courageously describes the evolution of the analyst's response to an analysand who cannot be reached. Boris forthrightly conveys the frustration in providing for a patient whose mind alternatively excites, challenges, and thwarts the analyst. Movement is countered by what Coltart calls "the mind back on duty."

What is needed to release the grip of the mind object? Stewart and Bollas underscore the importance of regression in the treatment of these cases, the frequency of sessions that facilitate this movement, as well as the resultant confusional states that must be born by patient and analyst. Bollas's patient is eventually released to a curative silence where he can rediscover maternal care and dependence. In the conjoint treatment of Simon and his mother, a holding environment was created that encouraged regressive forms of play and interaction where mother and baby could rediscover each other.

The necessity of the patient's experiencing the alive, human presence of a thinking, feeling analyst is highlighted in these essays. Eigen and the mystic battle for her soul as the analyst risks self exposure and vulnerability. Unencumbered by rigid technical rules, Bollas deftly and at times boldly shifts his stance with his troubled patient—actively intervening, quietly stepping back—in response to the patient's needs. Simon's analyst retains his vitality in the face of this young child's destructiveness and speaks to the buried truths of the child's desires.

In each case we view the sensitive provision of a particular kind of relationship. Just as the mind as omnipotent controller needs to be replaced by the mind as useful aide, so the all-knowing analyst must be replaced by the adaptively responsive participant. Then and only then can the patient find himself in the mind of another or as Boris puts it, "You think, therefore I am."

Peter Shabad and Stanley Selinger (Chapter 10) and Adam Phillips (Chapter 11) provide fitting closing chapters to this volume as they creatively reinterpret in their own very particular voices the theoretical issues first raised by Winnicott. Shabad and Selinger capture the infant's dilemma: "The baby compensates for who is not there by enclosing himself in a mental relationship with himself." These chapters are evocative as well as provocative essays as they carry implications beyond the patient to society as a whole and to the role of psychoanalysis in particular. Echoing Shabad's concern, Phillips asks, "What stops psychoanalytic theory (and practice) from becoming a mind object? . . . How can psychoanalysis keep the unknown in the picture?"

This collection of essays is an attempt to explore the dangers of knowing too much—the lure of the intellect—not only for the patient but for the analyst. They are meant to illuminate the complex pathological consequences that derive from precocious solutions and to provoke discussion of a neglected topic in psychoanalysis.

REFERENCES

Khan, M. (1971). Infantile neurosis as a false-self organization. In *Privacy of the Self*. New York: International Universities Press, 1974.
Winnicott, D. W. (1988). *Human Nature*. New York: Schocken.

1

The Mind as an Object

Edward G. Corrigan
Pearl-Ellen Gordon

CLINICAL OBSERVATIONS

In one extreme case an intellectual overgrowth that is successful in accounting for adaptation to need becomes of itself so important in the child's economy that it (the mind) becomes the nursemaid that acts as mother-substitute and cares for the baby in the child self. [*Human Nature*, Winnicott 1988, pp.139–140]

Mr. A., a 63-year-old self-made architect, whose "mind-set" as he puts it, has been "never to fail," tells his therapist, in an agonizing moment of recognition, "I am in fierce control. . . . The very act of making something happen—no matter how insignificant—is what it is about for me. . . . I must have always known that only I could do it. . . ."

Mr. B., a 55-year-old journalist, is far too busy to come to twice-a-week therapy. He prefers a single double-session to which he is invariably late. Actually, this mode of treatment suits him; slowly, over time, this intense, hyperactive man develops a capacity for reflection. In a key moment he tells his therapist, "My mind is like a factory, it has to produce work."

Miss C., an overweight, at times profoundly depressed, 40-year-old woman, has suffered two breakdowns. She speaks of never being able to relax or trust her academic and career accomplishments. Despite exemplary achievement, fears of failure and exposure are ever present. Every test is experienced as the first performance. For her, there are only two grades: "100% and 0." "I cannot rest on my laurels," she says. "There is never any peace . . . my life is work. Everything sticks to my mind . . . like contact paper."

Mrs. D., an engaging, 30-year-old physician, begins to review several recent decisions: marriage in her second year of medical school, a baby in her third year, a taxing, full-time job, the purchase of a large house, somewhat beyond her means. "I do everything in a hurry. . . . I'm always ahead of time . . . but I feel if I wait, it won't happen."

Sabrina, an 8-year-old, comes into the waiting room uncharacteristically arguing with her mother. Sullenly, she walks into her therapist's office. "I'm not going to the birthday party," she declares emphatically, her lips trembling as she fights back tears. Prodded by her therapist's questions, she slowly reveals the details. It is the birthday of one of her best friends, but she has lost the invitation and, therefore, cannot go. While she acknowledges that she can easily find out the time and place of the party, she insists that she has lost the invitation and therefore cannot attend. She stubbornly holds onto her strange logic. When her therapist says that she feels much more comfortable punishing herself for her mistakes than having others do it, which, parenthetically they did not and would not, her mood changes. She smiles and states that is "exactly right." "Now, you understand. Now you know why I can't go!"

Lily, a verbally facile, quite tall, but seriously overweight 6-year-old, plays at being an overburdened but uncomplaining Cinderella while her therapist is assigned the role of a querulous and demanding stepfather. A multitalented Cinderella can do anything and everything. She can clean a hundred bathrooms, complete a million chores a day. To quote Lily as Cinderella: "I was born 16. I never had diapers, never had a bottle, no pacifier, no thumb, no baby food."

Emma, a 5-year-old child described by Kerry Kelly (1970) in her paper, "A Precocious Child in Analysis," begins to crawl down the stairs very quickly and her analyst warns her, "Be careful, babies need help sometimes." Emma answers, "But it's not always there, so I manage by myself."

Sufficient unto their minds, gifted, it appears, intellectually or with a keen business savvy, some of our adult patients have achieved substantial, even extraordinary success, academically and financially. But as their treatment moves forward, Mr. A. and Mr. B. both wonder, what is life itself about? Has their life merely been a performance? Others, Mrs. C., for example, have suffered mental breakdown.

These patients vary in the nature and extent of their pathology as well as in personal style; some are narcissistic, some depressed, some boringly obsessive, while others are wonderfully quick and humorous. None of these patients are on particularly good terms with their instincts or with their bodies in general. Sexually, their symptomatology ranges from inhibition to perversity. Somatically, all of the adults we mentioned suffer from a variety of serious conditions: heart disease, gastrointestinal disorders, drug abuse, obesity, and anorexia. With respect to the children, Sabrina and Lily are overweight and Emma is enuretic. On psychological testing, many reveal startlingly high verbal IQs and only average performance IQ scores.

Significantly, their relationships lack expressiveness and spontaneity that can be sustained; our patients are actually quite dependent and controlling. Inevitably, they disappoint those whom they might initially captivate or impress. They cannot relax into just being, but must be constantly stimulated and enlivened by something or someone outside themselves. Yet, essentially fearful and negativistic, they do not surrender to any relationship and thus leave the other feeling useless.

In summary, we have come to view each of these patients as fiercely attached to their mind as an object, an object whose use is overvalued and exploited, whose existence is vigilantly protected, whose loss is constantly dreaded. Striving to disavow reliance on others, they have empowered the mind as the locus of self-holding and self-care. The mind object promises perfection and omnipotent control, but this ceaseless search never yields to satisfaction, only to anxiety, depression, and threatened breakdown.

LITERATURE REVIEW

We have found it useful to think of our patients who exploit their intelligence in the service of defense as exhibiting precocious ego development. How can ego development be premature? Why does ego development accelerate? What are the consequences of this unique skewing of development for the expression of drives, the sense of self, the quality of object relations? In this theoretical overview we shall explore these questions and highlight some of the special clinical issues and technical problems that confront the therapist treating the precocious patient.

Approaching the subject from different vantage points, various psychoanalytic writers have been intrigued by the notion of precocious development. Some have investigated the very gifted, talented, or creative child and focused on positive adaptation or the surmounting of developmental difficulties (Greenacre 1971). Others have looked more closely at specialness and fierce independence and found that the reliance on mind and the intellectual function at the expense of action and bodily experience can be a serious pathogenic factor in early development. The connection between precocity and obsessional neuroses can be found in the major psychoanalytical writings on the subject (Kulish 1988). Freud first suggested the link in a 1913 paper:

> I suggest the possibility that a chronological outstripping of libidinal development by ego development should be included in the disposition to obsessional neurosis. A precocity of this kind would necessitate the choice of an object under the influence of the ego-instinct, at a time which the sexual instincts had not yet assumed their final shape, and a fixation at the stage of pregenital sexual organization would thus be left. . . . [p. 325]

Anna Freud (1965) continued to speak of the pathological consequences of development proceeding at different speeds in different areas of the personality. Ego as relatively stronger than or more distant from drives is seen as the predisposing factor within the conflict model of obsessive-compulsive pathology. Nevertheless, the nature of the causative link is not clear, begging the question of whether precocious development is the cause or the effect. Does intelligence simply predispose to certain forms of illness or can it be exploited under certain kinds of circumstances?

What seems to be needed is a developmental perspective that goes beyond notions of psychic conflict and looks at the early interaction between innate endowment and environmental influence. Freud (1940) came closer to this in his paper on the splitting of the ego in the service of defense:

> I have at last been struck by the fact that the ego of a person whom we know as patient in analysis must, dozens of years earlier, when it was young, have behaved in a remarkable manner in certain particular situations of pressure. We can assign in general and somewhat vague terms the conditions under which this comes about by saying that it occurs under the influence of a psychical trauma. [p. 275]

Working on the same issue of trauma and its effect on the ego, Ferenczi has some intriguing thoughts on the patient whom he calls the "wise child." In his paper, "Confusion of Tongues," Ferenczi (1933) addresses the predicament of the child who is mistreated: "The weak or underdeveloped personality reacts to sudden unpleasure not by defense but by anxiety ridden identification and by introjection of the menacing person or aggressor" (p. 133). According to Ferenczi, the child enters into a traumatic trance through which he can deny the actuality of maltreatment, but at the expense of remaining confused and split. A precocious maturity is found in such children, "a traumatic progression." "Not only emotionally, but also intellectually can the trauma bring to maturity a part of the person" (p. 133).

In another paper entitled "Child-Analysis in the Analysis of Adults," Ferenczi (1931) vividly portrays the splitting of the self into a "suffering, brutally destroyed part and a part which knows everything but feels nothing" (p. 135). Ferenczi describes how in fantasies and dreams the patient expresses his split-off intelligence in the image of the head, "the organ of thought," cut off from the body, walking on its own feet or connected only by a thread. He cites in particular the typical dream of the "wise baby" in which a newborn or very young infant begins to talk or give sensible advice to its parents or other grown-ups. "The fear of the uninhibited, almost mad adult changes the child, so to speak, into a psychiatrist and in order to become one and to defend himself against the dangers coming from people without self control, he must know how to identify himself completely with them" (p. 135). We shall see how Ferenczi's ideas reverberate in the thoughts of D. W. Winnicott and Masud Khan. Parental failures, splitting of the ego, dissociation of affect, and the primacy of identification are central to our understanding of precocity.

It is to Winnicott's ideas especially and to Khan's creative elaborations that we have turned for our understanding of precocious development and conceptualization of the mind object.

Winnicott's theory of precocious development contains within it Freud's original observation of the "possibility of a chronological outstripping of libidinal development by ego development," but Winnicott expands upon Freud's insight in his own language, and in doing so, he vitalizes, both developmentally and clinically, the concept of premature ego development.

To begin with, Winnicott adds the mother to his theory, and then he places the baby in her holding environment. In health, this environment is at first "perfect"—the mother's adaptation to her infant is "very close to 100%"—and the infant's experience is of "going-on-being." But he adds that "it is a characteristic maternal function to provide *graduated failure of adaptation*, according to the growing ability of the individual infant to allow for relative failure by mental activity, or by understanding." To elaborate, "what releases the mother from her need to be near-perfect is the infant's understanding" (1949, p. 245).

But "if we take the case of a baby whose mother's failure to adapt is too rapid," Winnicott (1965a) writes in his paper, "New Light on Children's Thinking,"

> we can find that the baby survives by means of the mind. The mother exploits the baby's power to think things out and to collate and to understand. If the baby has a good mental apparatus this thinking becomes a substitute for maternal care and adaptation. The baby "mothers" himself by means of understanding, understanding too much. . . .
>
> This results in the uneasy intelligence of some whose good brains have become exploited. The intelligence is hiding a degree of deprivation. In other words, there is always for those with exploited brains a threat of a breakdown from intelligence and understanding to mental chaos or to disintegration of the personality. [p. 156]

In Winnicott's theory, "the psyche of the individual gets 'seduced' away into this mind from the intimate relationship which the psyche originally had with the soma" (1949, p. 247). The result is a "mind-psyche," located in the head, which is pathological, as there is no partnership between the mind-psyche and the body. Fiercely guarded will be what Adam Phillips (1988), in reviewing Winnicott, has described as a fantasy of self-sufficiency. The mind will be used not to continue mother's care, but to displace it altogether. According to Winnicott, a person who is developing in this way displays a distorted pattern affecting all later stages of development.

Khan (1963b) elaborated Winnicott's notion of maternal failure with his concept of cumulative trauma and its ego-biasing effects. Khan conceptualized precocious development as a consequence of the "silently and invisibly" accumulating breaches in the mother's role as a "protective shield." The infant becomes precociously aware of the mother as an object and must exploit whatever mental functions are available for self-defense.

Cumulative trauma has its beginnings in the period of development when the infant needs and uses the mother as his protective shield. The inevitable and temporary failures of the mother as protective shield are corrected and recovered from the evolving complexity and rhythm of the maturational processes. Where these failures of the mother in her role as protective shield are significantly frequent and lead to impingement on the infant's psyche-soma, impingements which he has no means of eliminating, they set up a nucleus of pathogenic reaction. These in turn start a process of interplay with the mother which is distinct from her adaptation to the infant's needs. [p. 53]

This negative interplay between mother and child can lead to premature and selective ego development, which can have several derailing effects on the development of a differentiated sense of self, on the vicissitudes of body ego development, and on the nature of the tie to objects.

The workings of the precocious ego can be quite elaborate, mystifying to the diagnostician, and often resistant to the usual interpretive efforts, as Khan (1971) establishes in his paper, "Infantile Neurosis as a False-Self Organization." Here he provides a different light on the connection between precocity and the obsessive-compulsive neurosis. Khan describes a man whose precocious mental development took over "the whole person of the child and militantly organized his internal world." Khan argues that "given a certain proclivity and endowment for premature ego development in response to traumata, there can be a precocious structuralization of the developmental process by acute dissociation and splitting leading to a false-self that we see retrospectively as an infantile neurosis of an obsessional kind" (p. 220). In this case what looked like an obsessional neurosis was not, in terms of classical theory, an intrapsychic achievement, but a false-self organization in response to early threats of annihilation of the psyche. An infantile neurosis was created through precocious exploitation of mental function. Winnicott understood this connection well, commenting that "intelligence can be exploited and . . . it can hide such things as deprivation and threatened chaos. A partial breakdown is represented by an obsessional organization, with disorganization always around the corner" (1989, pp. 156–157). Khan explored the ways his patient had filled the void, a "lacking expectable environment," by inventing a psychic structure of religious thoughts and rituals to which he could become rigidly and pervasively attached. We call this psychic structure the *mind object*.

Conceptualizing the mind object as a psychic structure that replaces the relationship to a real object leads to a discussion of narcissism and omnipotence. Herbert Rosenfeld's work on the psychopathology of narcissism sheds light on the working of the mind as object. He comments that "in narcissistic object relations omnipotence plays an important part" (1964, p. 170). Describing the variable structure of the narcissistic omnipotent self, Rosenfeld writes:

> Omnipotent phantasies may be stimulated during all phases from infancy to adulthood. None the less we have to remember that the omnipotent phantasies originated in infancy at a time when the individual felt helpless, small, and incapable of coping with the reality of being born and all the problems related to it. From birth onwards he not only built up a phantasy of an omnipotent self but also omnipotently created objects (at first part-objects) which would always be present to fulfil his desires. In this situation separation, overindulgence, or, particularly, the lack of a holding and containing environment increases the development and persistence of narcissistic structures. [1987, p. 87]

From our perspective, we would like to argue that the mind object is an omnipotently created object always available for mastery and control of internal objects so that dependence and the feelings it generates—anxiety, frustration, anger, and envy—can be obliterated. The mind object can be seen as a narcissistic, omnipotent organization, a personified force within, which over time exerts increasingly powerful influence, battling anything and anyone that threatens to expose it as illusionary.

Turning from adults to children, we find in the literature clinical examples of how precocity is set in motion. Martin James (1960), in his paper "Premature Ego Development: Some Observations on

Disturbances in the First Three Months of Life," provides us with an unusual window into the evolution of precocity, substantiating with infant observation the assertion that ego can indeed be premature. Presenting observations on a baby girl who was followed for seven years, James argues that constitutional influences, what we are accustomed to think of as givens, can be set in motion by an early noxious environment. The appearance and growth of autonomous functions are accelerated. A capacity for disappointment and delay in some "prodromal neural way" was forced on this infant who was in a state of hunger for the first three months of life. At two weeks of age this girl looked like a much older baby, more attentive and purposive, forced to tolerate delay; she exhibited signs that she was prematurely aware of her mother as an object. Perception and memory became overly and prematurely awakened. At three months when she was quiet she appeared bewildered, discouraged, and distressed. She revealed a range of negative affects that were precociously elaborated and uncommon to one so young. These feelings alternated with states of hyperactivity and hypersensitivity. Mental alertness and liveliness, fluidity of identification, and intellectual lopsidedness characterized her early childhood and were modified in some, but not all, respects by means of an enforced regression suggested to the parents by James when she was 2 years old. In following this girl James is quite aware of how a child can be pushed forward, the flight into the mind further exploited by parents who selectively respond to the child in terms of their own unconscious needs and fears. He warns:

> we may say that it is important to note how hard it may be for parents to resist the pressure and seduction of one sidedness in favor of all-round development. It is easy for the parent to take credit for having a forward child and not to notice at the time the loss of later ego-integration from narcissistic development not achieved through object relations. [1960, pp. 110–111]

What may evolve is a collusion between parent and child, both devoted to the maintenance and elaboration of specialness. The child becomes an object, a talented, gifted prize.

Kerry Kelly (1970) highlights the issues facing a child in analysis whose beginnings were not so traumatic as James's baby. Emma, a gifted child, developing speech and motility early, could be startlingly clever and observant. But too early she became aware of her mother's depressive, borderline character and her mother's continual demand that she be special. Weighing less than 5 pounds, Emma was born 6 weeks prematurely. The mother reported that Emma took easily to bottle feeding and was always a contented baby. She also insisted that she started Emma on solids at two weeks. "This is implausible and probably not true, but gives a picture of what Emma's mother wanted of her premature and particularly vulnerable infant" (p. 126).

In Khan's terms, we might say that for Emma, the maternal protective shield was precipitously pierced resulting in too early awareness of the object—too early Emma became sensitive to the unconscious needs of her depressed and disorganized mother.

There is a dreadful quality to Emma's awareness of her relation to her mother. Emma sadly reports, "Mommies get children to do things by frightening them." What, at some moments seems like charming sensitivity, at other moments reveals her inner sense of the actual, impossible dilemma she faces with her mother. In one session she explained to her therapist "the horriblest way to die." As Kelly describes, it occurs in a game where a witch and a fairy were struggling to kill each other. The witch had a plan to trick the fairy by first becoming friends with her. Then she would kill her. "Emma said this was the worst way to die because the fairy would not only be dead, she would be disappointed" (p. 126).

In a significant footnote, Kelly expands on the theme of disappointment and its relation to precocity.

> It was manifested in many ways, such as in her intense fear that adults would be disappointed in her, with the consequent desperate striving for precocious achievement, and the feeling that she was never good or grown up enough, but the most significant aspect lay in her manifold defenses against her own disappointment in her inadequate mother. Emma's prematurely developed reality testing gave way to blanket denial in the face of her conflicts over the sadness and re-

sentment aroused by her clear perception of her mother's problems
and failings. [p. 127]

Perhaps Winnicott might suggest that Emma, "tricked" or seduced into a precocious adaptation, has already suffered a death, a
psychic death. The collapse of the maternal holding environment
heralds the foreclosure of the generation of self-experience.

An observation from Adam Phillips (1993) aptly describes this
situation. He writes that "what Winnicott calls the False Self is invented to manage a prematurely important object. The False Self
enacts a kind of dissociated regard or recognition of the object; the
object is taken seriously, is shown concern, but not by a person"
(p. 34). Perhaps, we might say, that without treatment, Emma's
brittle precocity might have consolidated around the mind object—
"the false self located in the mind" (Khan 1969, p. 214)—but Emma
as an alive child connected to her wishes would be missing.

CENTRAL ANXIETIES AND DEFENSES AND
THEIR EFFECT ON OBJECT RELATIONS

When we consider these cases in the literature and our own work
with similar children and adults, we have been struck with several
unique problems faced by these patients. We can see, following
Winnicott and Khan, that once a precocious adaptation has been
set into play, it brings into its sphere of influence all further developmental experiences, resulting in specific kinds of twists and distortions. In Balint's terms, it represents a "basic fault."

All of our patients reveal central difficulties in the handling of
aggression. Khan speaks of the mystery of the transformation of
affects; we see violent rage—the rage of those whose aliveness has
been obliterated—become transformed into manic and precocious
ego functions. Put starkly, dissociated aggression fuels mind production. Mr. B. speaks of his mind as a factory. Lily rapidly produces page after page for a book whose bulk is more important than

its content. On the cover this precocious 5-year-old writes that she is author, copywriter, and illustrator. Young and old, our patients reveal the primitive workings of their superegos, which are also continually refueled by their anger. Identified with the aggressor, they brutally attack and criticize themselves. Severe and sadistic internal object relations predominate and shape superego formation. Furthermore, profound disillusionment in parents fosters the premature and rigid structuring of unalterable ego ideals. Having prematurely internalized parental standards, they expect too much from themselves, are often quite unrealistic, at times, omnipotent in their self-demands. The example of 8-year-old Sabrina denying herself a birthday party poignantly illustrates this. They are thus prey to intense feelings of anxiety, guilt, and inadequacy, which further enrages them and, in a vicious cycle, pushes them to more activity, more mind production. Perhaps when the mind attacks and brutalizes the self, we can speak of a superego precocity that goes hand and hand with ego precocity.

Identification with the aggressor is but one example of the pervasiveness of the defensive use of identification and imitation that patients exploit. Lily was a master at role playing significant powerful adults in her life—her parents, teachers, doctors. I was startled to feel her six-foot-four-inch father, who could be frighteningly enraged, emerge in the room. However, what seemed initially perceptive, clever, and engaging soon became repetitive and rigidly fixed. The script was written and neither she nor I could deviate. Describing his patient as a young girl, James explains that if she spent some time with other children, she quickly and fluidly picked up their mannerisms, speech, postures, and interests.

This particular child's character at five was full of attributions. Being with her, if one knew the quotations, was like listening to a musical pot-pourri. Socially, this passed as deliberate and to some was even an attraction. I think it could make us uneasy if we consider it a narcissistic process of identification and as such a substitute for true object relations. [1960, p. 108]

In dynamic terms, disillusionment and rage can be cleverly avoided
by the assumption of a "false identificatory oneness" (Khan 1963b,
p. 53). Khan elucidates:

> It is rather characteristic of reactive ego development and character
> formation that the patient is very much like the hero in Joyce's
> *Finnegans Wake*: "Here comes everybody." It is one of the results of
> the failure of personalization that the human being can be every-
> body and is a nobody. [1963a, p. 185]

With such heavy reliance on identification at the expense of real
object relating on the one hand and the ruthless assertion of self-
sufficiency on the other, these patients are severely compromised
in the development of a separate and coherent sense of self. So
strongly are they attached to their omnipotent inner objects that
they are blocked in internalizing new objects, in assimilating new
experiences. The stereotyped play of our child patients—Lily's insis-
tent repetition of the same roles—exemplifies this. Their negativity
toward an alive engagement with real people keeps them unconsciously tied to their primary objects. A dissociation occurs, as the
archaic maternal object and the fantasies that surround her remain
unintegrated. While a pseudo-independence is asserted and mind
production fueled, as Khan (1963) explains, "an archaic dependency
bond is exploited" (p. 54).

Our child patients can be extremely controlling and demanding,
even oppressive at times. Lily's father, who could extol on the brilliance of his daughter, compared her to Hannibal Lechter, the can-
nibalistic psychiatrist in *The Silence of the Lambs*.

In our adult patients, whose defenses are more elaborated, this
dissociated dependence is expressed more subtly. Mr. B. was in a
constant state of frenzy in his office, involved in many activities that
he felt only he could handle. A young and inept assistant was rele-
gated to doing all the unimportant busy work. Mr. B. was demanding and exploitative of him, critical and contemptuous of his often
disorganized efforts. For years he talked of firing him, but did noth-

ing. The needy, vulnerable parts of Mr. B. had been projected into this inept assistant, and thus Mr. B. lived out his dissociated dependency needs at the same time as he railed against them. Coming home at night he would tell his wife endless tales of his day. He relied on her constant presence but was never able to acknowledge this need or comprehend her anger and disappointment at not being related to in an alive and mutual way. As a result of this unspoken dependence on one hand and self-reliance on the other, our patients are often beset by profound feelings of loneliness. We have heard dream images of being "above it all," images that convey both their solution and their dilemma.

Clearly, our patients do not feel connected to or alive in their bodies. In a sense they are heads without bodies. This was dramatically and visually proclaimed in the case of Miss C., whose beautiful face emerged from a large formless and often unkempt body, and in the case of Mrs. D., whose round face with huge, alive eyes emerged in the early stages of treatment from a short, painfully thin stick of a body. As we have indicated, we see fixations, inhibitions, and perversions in adult patients as uneven ego development distorts the evolution of libidinal stages. The children seem to rely on infantile modes of need satisfaction: thumb sucking, masturbation, nail biting, compulsive eating. Often, with parental collusion, they can be quite secretive about these habits, some of which are only recognized as treatment progresses. On the one hand, expressing intolerance of babyish needs and vulnerabilities, Lily complained of how silly the little girls in her class were. On the other hand, a compulsive nail biter and eater, she was whiny and demanding of constant attention at home. For some of our patients their bodies are felt as persecutors and are treated in the way they experienced their mothers treating them. Lily continually reenacted her parent's sadistic handling of the feeding situation. Starved as an infant because her mother was afraid she would grow fat as she had done, Lily had become an overweight child, unable to regulate intake and harshly critical of her body. Mrs. D. in young adulthood had become seriously anorexic, massively denying the withering away of her body to the extent that it was a painful experience for her to sit in the leather chair in the therapist's office.

What our patients do cathect is their mind. For some patients, the mind object, dominating and attacking, is at odds with the self. For others, adoring and aggrandizing, it is at one with the self. Nevertheless, enemy or ally, the mind object has for our patients an independent and powerful existence. They are attached to its inner workings—to their unusual capacities to apprehend external reality as well as, for some, their propensity to spin forth internal fantasy. For many patients, there are times when there is real pleasure in the use of the mind, indeed there may even be a sense of triumph. Consciously, they have succeeded, produced, achieved, dazzled; unconsciously, they celebrate their capacity for survival in the face of the annihilating object. For some, this pleasure can last a long time; we must remember that precocity is a disorder of adaptation much valued in our culture.

Most of our patients, however, are preoccupied with the state of their mind. It is difficult for such patients not to know and yet patients who rely on their mind as an object, on some level, actually know all too well of its unreliability. Speaking of children, Winnicott writes: "There is nothing that a child can do about being held by a split off function except to think of the mechanics of its working well or badly" (1965b, p. 160). Our patients often complain of being dumb and stupid. On the one hand, they are fearful of losing control; on the other, they may be unconsciously aware of their false self adaptation, of the distortion of the true function of their minds. Such complaints may conceal powerful wishes to be "mindless." Nonetheless, they fiercely defend their mindful state. It was impossible to teach Lily anything—she needed to know it all; she insisted that she knew it all! Lily refused to engage in board games. Precocious children play games they can win. While competitiveness is an issue, more central seems to be their unwillingness to acknowledge they need to be taught how to play. To experience not knowing is far too dangerous; safety and security reside in the mind as object.

THE TREATMENT DILEMMA

Why do such patients come for treatment? What are they seeking, consciously and unconsciously? As we have argued, if the mind as object is working well, there is little need for the other. Thus our patients come for help when there is some threat of breakdown of their defense. For example, in children, this is seen at developmental stress points, particularly at times of increased separation from mother, when they cannot sustain the dissociation of their archaic dependency needs. School, where they often can perform quite brilliantly, presents them with social demands that can feel overwhelming. They cannot match their perfectionistic ideals. With the adults, we often find the presenting problems revolve around an increasingly problematic relationship. Interpersonal demands and possible abandonment threaten their intrapsychic balance and their need for omnipotent control and for an aura of self-sufficiency. In older patients, a nagging feeling of hopelessness and emptiness may haunt them, and they come to treatment with a particular kind of despair.

Nonetheless, these are not easy patients to treat as they put the therapist in the paradoxical position of offering help to someone who essentially needs to disclaim help. They have long ago assumed the role of private psychic nurse. With our patients, child and adult, we have encountered difficult and perplexing transference and countertransference dilemmas, many of them organized around the patient's need for mental control with which we can all too easily and unwittingly collude. With some patients for whom everything seems to be working well, we interpret and the patient may respond brilliantly. Indeed, we often consider these patients special in the quick way they take to the analytic agenda. We are pleased with the treatment—we appear to be a "perfect" analytic couple, that is, until the patient suddenly brings the treatment to a premature end, perhaps after a separation during which their dependency feelings might have emerged, however dimly. Having achieved, in relative terms, their conscious goal in the treatment—repaired self-sufficiency—they depart or cut back on the frequency of sessions. Coldly, they leave us without turning back. We feel shut out, let down, not knowing what hit us. We are unprepared for their exit, because, aside from subtle countertransference warnings, our patients have rarely expressed direct aggression toward us.

Rather, our patients have many clever strategies for avoiding disappointment and anger. We have observed their often impressive caretaking capacities of others, including ourselves. They are masters of spotting dependent and primitive longings and, quickly identifying with the active role, they take charge to help and repair (Winnicott 1949). With ease and understanding, they change hours to suit the therapist's convenience. Many deny problems with vacations. Smiling warmly, one young adult exclaimed, "You know, I'm one of those who never miss you over the summer." Expression of dissociated feelings takes place outside of the analytic sessions. Miss C. missed many sessions due to repetitive illnesses. Somatizing her dependent longings, she took to her bed, ate, and watched TV. Mrs. D. had an intense extramarital affair for months before telling her therapist. Intolerant of his own vulnerability, Mr. A. belittled and humiliated his homosexual son for being ineffectual. With these maneuvers, real dependence, the experience of which would return them to the maternal space within the transference where they would, no doubt, experience many disorganizing and frightening affects, is skillfully dodged for long periods of time. Indeed, for many, it is never entered.

Some patients reveal vivid memories of the past and have become precise recorders and catalogers of their experience. Others have a singular gift for auto-interpretation (Green 1986). The play of precocious children can appear singularly inventive, zeroing in on central dynamics with astonishing precision. Lily enacted the compliant, uncomplaining patient to my sadistic doctor or the supergifted, everdutiful Cinderella for whom no task was too large to my petulant, demanding stepfather. But her play proved to be boringly repetitive and stultifyingly rigid. With precocious patients, the sense of the session is frequently not of an enriching free associative elaboration, but of defensive control in the service of knowing it all.

In our countertransference with some of these patients, we can ourselves feel dumb and useless, with nothing to say. It is as if we are holding that part of the patient that he needs to dissociate. One child patient was repeatedly playing a board game and mercilessly beating her opponent with strokes of amazing genius. The therapist gave voice, in a somewhat humorous way, to feeling absolutely hopeless and defeated with respect to the game. The child told her with utter contempt to stop whining or she would tell her parents to stop paying her. Nonetheless, her arrogant control modified slightly as the session progressed. With a more disturbed patient, the analyst can, at times, feel utterly obliterated by the patient's exclusive use and abuse of his or her own mind; in our counter-transference we are thrown back into the patient's early environment where his or her nascent being was destroyed. We find that the analytic use of silence as a medium for reflection unnerves some patients and they often head it off with their own self-analysis, self-criticism, or obsessive repetition, all of which eventually render us blank and impotent, without associative response. The use of language itself can provide the patient with a powerful tool to keep us distant and affect-blunted. In the countertransference, we find ourselves, uncannily, offering up our own premature interpretations. In so doing we may surprise and terrify the patient with the thought that someone knows more than he or she does. Competitiveness, envy, a too-easy dismissal may be generated. Unwittingly, we may be drawn into repeating the original trauma in creating an overly demanding analytic situation. In doing so we subtly reinforce the patient's unconscious feelings of disappointment and despair.

While it is difficult to resist the seduction of the intellect and the mental gamesmanship that can get going, we do not want to support the patient's style of self-defense. One walks a thin tight-rope (Coltart 1992) in not doing this, as precocious patients also require an appreciative audience and a ready intelligence in the therapist. What the patient needs is a personal relationship with another who can risk not knowing, who can bear uncertainty, who can fumble and recover, who can be wrong and be comfortable with difference (Khan 1974). To insure this, the whole analytic setting, the therapeutic environment, and its reliable maintenance become of central importance. Winnicott and Khan describe how the patient is unconsciously looking for a relationship with an object who will both carefully protect the conditions necessary for growth and provide an affectively alive responsiveness to a highly sensitive and perceptive psyche.

We have been struck by the importance of ordinary regressions, as when the precocious adult is able to lie quietly and contentedly or when the child becomes silly and playful, when there is lightness, humor, and pleasure in the analytic atmosphere or when there is sadness that is not quickly dismissed. At these times we become aware of a body in the room as well as a mind. Held by the therapist and the therapeutic setting, the patient may be able to release the tight grip of the mind object. Eventually, he may be able to re-experience, regressively and affectively, in the transference, what Khan (1960) calls the "total fragmentary reality that he has been carrying around under magical control" (p. 25). However, while we may strive to sustain our own aliveness and maintain the conditions that facilitate the regressive process, the precocious child or adult tenaciously holds to the relationship to the mind object—an object that can be idealized and adored as well as vilified, an object that can protect and enliven as well as tyrannize. Foward movement in treatment is often disavowed and negated in future sessions; the precocious patient proves singularly difficult to treat. The mind object is a bossy advisor, a seductive friend to the patient but a fearsome competitor, a hostile saboteur to the therapist. Eventually, the patient's underlying despair can be matched by our own.

We will bring our discussion to a close by citing a critical statement of Winnicott's (1971) that appears in his introduction to *Playing and Reality*. There, while asking his readers to accept the paradox involved in the infant's use of the transitional object, he points out that "by the flight to split-off intellectual functioning, it is possible to resolve the paradox, but the price of this is the loss of the value of the paradox itself" (p. xii). From Winnicott's point of view, the loss of the paradox implied in the use of the transitional object through premature intellectual functioning indicates the loss of intermediate space, playing, and creativity. We suggest that the mind object—an object of intense attachment—substitutes for a transitional object and subsumes intermediate phenomena to its domain. But the mind as an object is an illusion. The clinical task is to reestablish the intermediate area as the place where life is lived—where there can be delight in the use of the mind that is expressive and mutual.

REFERENCES

Coltart, N. (1992). *Slouching Towards Bethlehem*. London: Free Association.
Ferenczi, S. (1931). Child-analysis in the analysis of adults. In *Problems and Methods of Psycho-Analysis*, ed. M. Balint. New York: Brunner/Mazel, 1980.
—— (1933). Confusion of tongues between adults and the child. In *Problems and Methods of Psycho-Analysis*, ed. M. Balint. New York: Brunner/Mazel, 1980.
Freud, A. (1965). *Normality and Pathology in Childhood: Assessments of Development*. New York: International Universities Press.
Freud, S. (1913). The predisposition to obsessional neurosis. *Standard Edition*. 12:311–326.
—— (1940). Splitting of the ego in the process of defence. *Standard Edition*. 23:275–278.
Green, A. (1986). *On Private Madness*. New York: International Universities Press.
Greenacre, P. (1971). *Emotional Growth: Psychoanalytic Studies of the Gifted and a Great Variety of Other Individuals*. New York: International Universities Press.
James, M. (1960). Premature ego development: some observations on disturbances in the first three months of life. In *The British School of Psychoanalysis: The Independent Tradition*, ed. G. Kohon. New Haven: Yale University Press, 1986.
Kelly, K. (1970). A precocious child in analysis. *Psychoanalytic Study of the Child*. 25:122–145. New York: International Universities Press.
Khan, M. (1960). Clinical aspects of the schizoid personality: affects and technique. *In Privacy of the Self*. New York: International Universities Press, 1974.
—— (1963a). Ego-ideal, excitement, annihilation. In *Privacy of the Self*. New York: International Universities Press, 1974.
—— (1963b). The concept of cumulative trauma. In *Privacy of the Self*. New York: International Universities Press, 1974.
—— (1969). Vicissitudes of being, knowing and experiencing in the therapeutic situation. In *Privacy of the Self*. New York: International Universities Press, 1974.

—— (1971). Infantile neurosis as a false-self organization In *Privacy of the Self.* New York: International Universities Press, 1974.

—— (1974). *The Privacy of the Self.* New York: International Universities Press.

Kulish, N. (1988). Precocious ego development and obsessive compulsive neurosis. *Journal of the American Academy of Psychoanalysis.* 16(2):167–187.

Phillips, A. (1988). *Winnicott.* Cambridge, MA: Harvard University Press.

—— (1993). *On Kissing, Tickling and Being Bored: Psychoanalytic Essays on the Unexamined Life.* Cambridge, MA: Harvard University Press.

Rosenfeld, H. (1964). On the psychopathology of narcissism: a clinical approach. In *Psychotic States.* London: Karnac.

—— (1987). *Impasse and Interpretation.* London: New Library of Psychoanalysis.

Winnicott, D. W. (1949). Mind and its relation to the psyche-soma. In *Through Paediatrics to Psycho-Analysis.* New York: Basic Books, 1975.

—— (1965a). New light on children's thinking. In *Psycho-Analytic Explorations.* Cambridge, MA: Harvard University Press, 1989.

—— (1965b). Comment on Obsessional Neurosis and "Frankie." In *Psycho-Analytic Explorations.* Cambridge, MA: Harvard University Press, 1989.

—— (1971). *Playing and Reality.* New York: Basic Books.

—— (1988). *Human Nature.* New York: Schocken.

—— (1989). *Psycho-Analytic Explorations.* Cambridge, MA: Harvard University Press.

2

A Philosopher and His Mind

Nina Coltart

In 1967, a man was referred to me by a colleague for five times a week psychoanalysis. Here is the first paragraph of the notes of my consultation with him exactly as I wrote it then; it still seems as vivid a picture of the man I slowly came to know so well as I would ever have written at any point since. "An eccentric individual. He arrived sweating, smelly, untidy, and slightly late, and launched descriptively into his recent psychiatric life, with many strange grimaces and odd tremors in his voice, betraying, I suppose, anxiety. His long gray hair floated randomly about his face and head. One might have guessed his occupation from his appearance and manner; he is a University Reader in Philosophy."

For some reason, and very unusually for me—I think because I continually found him so intractable and so strange—I kept notes on the analysis, a few lines per session, for almost all of the six years he was with me. It was an extraordinary event to read through this man's whole analysis; the notes included a number of letters from him, once when he worked at an American university for six months, and once when he ruptured his Achilles tendon and had to be in hospital for a few weeks. The reading took about eight hours altogether. The atmosphere of the analysis was strongly conveyed; sometimes I experienced a distinctly claustrophobic sense of it, which I did then remember feeling during individual sessions. Constant obsessional ruminations about his sleep pattern (insomnia was his main presenting symptom), exact details of his medication, and minute particulars of how he felt, psychically and physically, all combined to exert a monotonous, grinding pressure on me, the implicit—and sometimes explicit—message being: "*Do* something." But the message contained a deadly double bind, to which I shall return.

Careful study of the notes on the consultation, or preliminary session, reveals (as it so often does) a great deal of information and material of potential significance about this eccentric and deeply neurotic man. He was 43 when he came to me. He had recently terminated, against the analyst's advice, nine years of twice-weekly therapy with a male analyst considerably older than himself. He complained of three main things in respect of that treatment. He lay on the couch, and he always felt deprived of contact and response: he said he would get so frustrated that he "felt like kicking Dr. X"— but added "of course, I'm a coward about anger; I can't express it, though that's nothing to do with politeness." He added firmly that he was not going to lie on the couch here; unless he could see me, he was going elsewhere until he found an analyst who allowed it. I did not feel strongly about the point, as it happened, and I agreed that he should sit up.

Then he said there had been no transference work in his previous treatment, and he regarded that as a real failure. Of course he belonged to an intellectual class that knew a great deal about psychoanalysis, its theory and techniques. Furthermore, he had had earlier encounters with it in his life. I must admit that he seemed to offer plenty of material appropriate to transference work, and this was proved to be the case during analysis, although using it with a sense of authentic encounter was more problematical.

Finally, he complained that Dr. X had "generously offered" prescriptions for any amount of whatever drug he, the patient, wanted. This was typical of what turned out to be a knack, in the patient, for the ambivalent double binding of others; I have no doubt he twisted Dr. X's arm to prescribe for him in a way his own physician refused to do. Then he complained that Dr. X gave him far too much (by what he considered normal standards; he himself wanted it).

And he also expressed distaste for being able to control the analyst so easily. It was a lesson in the unwisdom of being particularly "kind" to patients, I thought. The drugs referred to were sedatives and hypnotics, with the occasional antidepressant thrown in.

He told me quite a lot about his family and early life, with a certain practiced fluency. He was the younger by four years of two brothers. He did not like, or enjoy the company of, his brother, who was married with two teenage children. His father was a Ukrainian Jew, and "an intellectual who failed to be a genius, and wanted me to be one instead; by now he is 75, a clown and a sneerer." His mother, then also 75, was "a dominating, powerful, cold, and imperceptive woman, with strong imposing views." The patient said, with concentrated venom: "I hate her more than anyone in the world." Nevertheless, he visited the parents every Sunday. I should add here that he lived alone, and although he was mean in his attitudes to other people, his own apartment was very expensive. He had been greatly favoritized as a child, over the brother. He had idealized his father until his teens, he said, but more importantly, he had realized that both parents had idealized *him*, sharing their hope and ambition—and for a long time, belief—that he was a genius. He made it clear that he had been idealized because of the entertaining brilliance of his mind and speech, his quaint perceptions, and his amusing and penetrating comments on life—all this from a very young age. He went to a special school run by Susan Isaacs, a Kleinian analyst, who had since written a book based on the school, called *The Intellectual Growth of the Child*; in this book, the patient was frequently quoted verbatim and he brought it to show me. I made it clear that it sufficed for him to tell me about it. He added: "But I am not a genius." There was an extraordinary quality to this remark; on the one hand, it was said in such a way as to suggest there might be room for doubt; on the other, there was a pathetic and sad resignation about it.

With a certain boldness arising out of giving this self-picture, the patient, whom I will call John, told me (a) that he required me to be very intelligent, (b) that he expected to be given extra time if he needed it—"as Dr. X always had," and (c) that he expected me to

medicate him according to his own demands. I responded briskly
that I would certainly not be complying with either (b) or (c) and
that I supposed (a) would be revealed, or not, soon enough. He put
his head to one side, and gave a strange smile and grimace; I read
it as partly annoyed and partly relieved.

The sessions began the following week; the early ones were devoted to trying to impress me with the quality of his mind, which
rapidly began to feel to me as if it should have a capital M. He also
spent time demonstrating to me how much he already understood
about his psychopathology, and striving to block any possible entry
of mine by formulating psychoanalytic insights, mingled with philosophical language. In a disaffected way, he related various sexual
fantasies to me, featuring sadomasochism. He explained to me that
he "tended to a Berkeleian view of absence"! Fortunately I knew a
couple of limericks that I thought summarized adequately such
knowledge of Berkeley as I might need.

> There was a young man who said: "God
> Must think it exceedingly odd
> That this old oak-tree
> Continues to be,
> When there's no-one about in the quad.

> Dear Sir: Your astonishment's odd;
> I am *always* about in the quad,
> And that's why this tree
> Continues to be
> Observed by yours faithfully, God.

I did not quote these limericks to John, partly because I imagined
that he knew them already. Nor did I ever just accept statements of
his that were clothed in philosophical concepts, but would ask him
to explain what he meant in ordinary language. I thought that accepting them as if I understood them (even when I did) would be
colluding with him in a game that would make us seem especially
clever, and would separate us in a conspiratorial union above the
mass of lesser brains who were comparatively stupid or ill-educated.

He told me, when speaking of his parents, that his mother was "very keen that he should get better," a remark that was later revealed as containing violent and vengeful fantasy on his part. It was also connected with the double bind on me to which I said I would return, and I will now describe it. He had to appear, and I thought that this was consciously true, as if he wanted to "get better" himself, else why was he here? And would I expend any effort on him if he did not want to, or even if he was ambivalent? Yet at the same time, in wishing to be better, he was aligning himself entirely with his mother and the conscious manifestation of *her* wish; this was anathema to him. His symptoms, particularly his chronic insomnia and his social unease, were also his powerful weapons in his life-long vengeful battle with her; and furthermore, the transference to me was, as a direct result of this double bind, extremely conflictual. It seems almost strange to me now, but early on in his analysis, none of this was conscious to him; and it was only through minutely detailed dissection of the transference that it all became clearer, and the connections were made between his hatred of his mother, the use of his disturbances as a weapon, and the negative undercurrents in the transference. He had said he wanted transference work, but when it came, he did not like it, and resisted it strongly; probably he had done so with some success in his previous therapy, and I surmised that then it was also much more opaque with a male analyst, and perhaps less intense.

This work also led into an exploration of one of his ways of relating to his mind as an object. A deeper conflict than that which had thus far colored the transference to me lay in a fixation to a development stage when he was 3 years old and (using Kohutian theory here) had been at his most narcissistically grandiose, particularly in his expectations that the precocious power of his mind was sufficient to conquer anyone, whatever the subject under discussion. By "conquer" it transpired that he meant that significant adults would, if there were arguments or attempts to control, or even teach him, quite rapidly give in to his way of seeing something, or his wish to do something, with apparent admiration and a meaningful exchange of glances (which he would watch for), as if to say, or so he thought: "Of course he's right—he's so clever we must yield to his judgment, he knows best." I imagine, if glances were exchanged, it was more likely that they were accompanied by a resigned sigh, and a view that although he was "adorable" because of his precocity, his will had become so strong (i.e., they had already "spoiled" him so much) that it was more than they cared to do to embark on a prolonged battle with him.

The deep conflict in his relationship to his mind at this stage, therefore, consisted in a persistent grandiose conviction that he was truly omnipotent, which, however, was chronically contaminated, or so it felt to him, by a recognition that he was not. He did not trust the admiring love of his internalized objects, because he had also correctly perceived in their "giving in" to him a weary anger, an impatience, a withdrawal of love, a coldness, and an absolutely certain knowledge that if they could trouble to exert themselves they could overrule his stubborn precocity. He therefore, in his final, and most unconscious self-awareness, did not trust his parents' love for him *nor* the power of his mind; and this was deeply distressing and depressing. One could, with some accuracy, say that they practiced a sort of double bind on him; that is, under their submissive, but genuine, admiration, they were also angry, critical, and anxious about him. He had become profoundly conditioned to believing he was loved and cared for only *on account of* his brilliance, and the subtle and amazing thoughts and words his mind was capable of. He had no hope at all that if he was silly and naughty, or, worse, infantile, full of rage and tantrums, and "boring" (a terrible label of contempt and dismissiveness from both his parents), he would be loved, looked after, and forgiven just the same, He would therefore desperately redouble his efforts to exert omnipotence, and in so doing, I guessed though he did not say, become more obnoxious and isolated; and this behavior had persisted until the time when I came to know him.

Most of this, I can deduce from my notes, was worked on endlessly and thoroughly, usually clothed in classical theory and language, which was nearly all that was available, at least to me, at the time. The result often seems to me now to be clumsy and my interpretations not "experience-near," as Kohut would say. It is much easier now to formulate ideas about John's very early life than it was then. But with the help of the transference and faithfully following its guidance, and the early writings of Winnicott, it seems that quite a lot that was really important about him and where and why he was stuck got conveyed.

I would like to consider for a moment the way in which Winnicott's concepts of True Self/False Self applied to this patient. Certainly a large proportion of his analysis was concerned with working on the sort of thing that these ideas summarized. Aphoristically, I could say of the psychopathology of the patient, "his mind ruined his life." It is probably accurate that in some people extreme self-consciousness accompanies, or is even a synonym for, the False Self. Furthermore, the self-conscious mind is the creator and organizer of the False Self. To be watched, ideally, in fantasy, with loving admiration, was such an important condition of John's early precocity that he was controllingly identified with the watcher, and in adult life could not escape from the split and the subsequent state of mind that this implies. Of course, we all, to some degree, create, and live conventionally in the world, through a False Self; the True Self, in essence, is, as Lacan points out, truly unconscious, made up of the elements of primary process, random and strong. But it is the source of all energy, and "genuine" people show in expressive living that they are much more in touch with this source. If we define the True Self as capable of originating natural, spontaneous, "first-hand" emotion and behavior, then we are bound to see that John's self-experience and self-description were undoubtedly those of a False Self. He felt incapable of the sort of genuineness and cathexis of objects that he thought, rightly, were implied by "natural" and "spontaneous." He was almost perpetually conscious of the splits whereby he was the watcher of his mind, and the performer, and the organizer. The performance, tragically, was of "*living.*" On one occasion, he cried, in a way which was for a moment an expression of authentic anguish: "I've forgotten how to act myself"; not even ". . . *be* myself," but, such was his parlous and despairing state, ". . . *act* myself." John wrote a lot of poetry and sometimes quoted it to me. One of his poems, which had real feeling in it, began: "The tragedy fell flat . . ." It went on to reveal that, after all, there was no audience—the actor was alone.

It was, he knew, his mind that betrayed him; it seemingly had a Midas touch. The story of King Midas, who wished for the ability to turn things that he touched to gold and had his wish granted, is one of grimness and horror, leading only to death. In John's case, if ever for a few moments he "forgot" himself and expressed, even *experienced*, a true firsthand emotion, his mind would instantly be back on duty, watching and dehumanizing his self. And yet it was this mind that he also continued to idealize, admire, rely on, and use in his "precocious" attempts to seduce and impress the world. One of his gifts, and it was extraordinary, was a memory-store of long poems and huge quantities of Shakespeare; any poem or passage that took his fancy could be absorbed in a relatively short time and quoted on the slightest appropriate occasion. I thought that the sense of disappearing inside the thoughts and language of another must be a rest from the ever-vigilant, exhausting job of living his own life, in an apparently sane way, from morning until night.

Night, of course, would relentlessly come, and with it John's major presenting symptom—insomnia. If there was one way that John apparently wanted to "get better," more than anything else it was that he wanted his insomnia cured. Everybody who knew John at all well was aware of him being insomniac. His parents were especially aware of it. He treated passing social inquiries as to how he was as questions about how he was sleeping. He very speedily took to giving me a detailed report on the previous night as an introduction to every session. John lived alone, but every Sunday, as I mentioned earlier, he visited his parents for tea; he hated his mother and disliked and despised his father, but he was still attached, dependent, and vengeful. He would say he went out of duty, and because they were elderly and they wanted him, but this shallow bluff did not deceive even him, although to begin with he denied his dependency and the other reason I thought was paramount, which was to demonstrate regularly to them that he was *not* "getting better," and so carry on his vengeful war of attrition. His mother made it clear that it would bring her real happiness if John could convey news of peaceful sleep; she rightly saw that this would entail much else— reduction in anxieties, increase in enjoyment of life. So this, with stubborn grimness, and at deep and lasting cost to his well-being, John refused to provide. It is a bitter affliction in life to use oneself as one's weapon in an ongoing war whose origins are lost in time and irretrievable by memory.

I will not go into the details of his insomnia; suffice it to say that he very rarely had a night of "natural" sleep; he took vast quantities of mixed medications sometimes twelve to fifteen tablets a night, and had various doctors and doctor-friends contributing to his stores, all unbeknownst to each other. It is of greater interest in this context to try to see how his mind treated sleeping as its own primary and singular object; sleep itself had become an impossibly idealized state whose secret function, among others, was to disappoint him and let him down, as did he and his mind to anyone who had high hopes of him and it. Similarities with how he had experienced his parents, especially his mother, as he grew up, were also evident. The insomnia had that particular resistance to analysis that is characteristic of a symptom that is, by definition, always outside the range of direct transference analysis. We were always talking *about* it, rather than it informing our talk. Gradually it became clearer how overdetermined it was, which again increased its resistant power; like the many-headed hydra, it could flourish to fight another day, even when one of its meanings could be so extensively understood that it might have lost strength through familiarity, if not through mutative interpretation.

Paradoxically, although he felt he ought to be able to "think himself" asleep, sleep was dreaded as a loss of control by the mind. John believed, in a way, and obstinately against much evidence to the contrary, that he *had* such control over his self in everyday life, but even though his mind would work ingeniously at ways of trying to get him to sleep, it seemed that the sense of escape into the unknown made these efforts ultimately and paradoxically frightening. It was as if he might disappear and never come back. In spite of a fascinated and serious preoccupation with suicide and death as the

only answer to his existential problems, it seemed that there was
not an exact parallel between death and sleep, which remained an
object of dread in a way that death did not. Sleep represented a
merging with mother and a loss of self; this meaning came up in
connection with associations to the story of Hansel and Gretel; John
did have a genuine intellectual curiosity and he could understand
how the children were driven forward by a similar curiosity into
the depths of the woods, and then led to trying to eat bits of the
sugar-and-gingerbread house; but this brought the terrifying old
witch who said she would eat *them*. In spite of the fact that John
had a fantasy that he would have been saved by what Kohut calls
the "merger transference," he was far too wary and self-conscious
to let it come about. He was, unconsciously, too afraid that I would
eat him.

Sleep also, to John's controlling mind, stood for something that
he ought to be able to *learn* how to do. But there was a severe and
early fracture in his ability to learn, which forever after contaminated the process. During the early stages of learning, and this went
right back to his first days at school when he was a precocious
3-year-old, he was found to be exceptionally bright. For a short while,
he would learn with ease—English, French, Latin, mathematics.
Then, rather suddenly, he would become less achieving; his unusual
capacities seemed to fade, and thereafter they never regained their
starry quality, although new subjects produced the same phenomenon and then followed the same downhill curve. Apart from his
remarkable "learning by heart" of poetry and drama, learning anything was a struggle and a disappointment to him all through his
life. He *was* very intelligent, and his learning was still at a higher
level than most people's, but he always found it hard and was always
dismissive of what he could do when compared to what he dimly
hoped for. For example, he got a First in philosophy, but was at a
university where sometimes "Starred Firsts" were given, and of
course that was what he should have had. Sleep became, as it were,
a Starred First. Furthermore, the complication of a sour envy of
those few who could and did do better than he came into the picture, and made his own experience of learning more fraught and

unhappy. I concluded that John was a person "wrecked by success" (Freud 1916). A perpetuation of his brilliant learning level would have represented the final failure of his secret hope that he could be loved for himself alone, his greedy, smelly, infantile self, and not for his miraculous mind.

A word about dreams. Whether it was a function of his high levels of self-observing consciousness to keep dreams at bay, I could never decide. But John dreamed very rarely, and when he did, the amount of secondary-process elaboration they received on their journey from him to me was such that I hardly ever felt a sense of conviction when trying to create some interpretation.

One way and another, through experience, I realized that the whole business of sleep had to be crept up on from some unexpected quarter, so that John and his mind were, so to speak, tricked into a yielding of his addiction to insomnia. After about three years of analysis, when his ability to express emotion as part of a conscious fantasy was more genuine, I began to notice that if he could express aggressive feeling *at* me, he slept better for several nights. At first his ways of doing it were tentative and indirect. For example, I observed, after a long time, that there could occur a deadly monotony in certain series of sessions, which I experienced as pressurizing, aggressive, and difficult to bear; he would go on and on about what I have noted as "a dreary, heavy, sadistically colored sequence of breasts, sleep, shit, breasts, sleep, shit!" I would interpret the low-grade continuous level of attack, and he might then step it up a bit; if I could only *help* him to do something to get *over* his obsessional thinking, then he might be able to *stop*, but I *wanted* his thoughts as they *came*, didn't I? In such ways he often tried to expose and shame me for not being as good at my work as I thought I was and for my self-satisfaction in the very presence of my deficiency and inadequacy.

From the rather anal fixation level of some of his thinking, he suffered quite markedly from shame, or the anticipation of shame, especially socially, and he tried all sorts of ways of displacing this into me. However, although he would sleep better, he found this aggressive behavior in himself quite difficult to tolerate for a long

time, although it gradually became more fluent; it caused him to
fall in his own grandiose self-esteem (one of his delusional self-
attitudes), and he felt he could only be raised again if I not only
made it clear that I cared uniquely for him, but also that I forgave
him for what he had done (and wanted to do) to me. When I would
not, but described what he was up to, made a transference interpretation, or remained silent, he became frantic and demanding,
and then elaborated a fantasy of blissful reconciliation and reunion,
in which he tended and cared for my injuries—caused by him, of
course. This is a particular slant that I have almost always come
across in people who use sadomasochism as characterological behavior. In turn the images of reconciliation would be followed by
quite viciously sadistic fantasy, which had then to be expiated, often
by increase in anxieties and return to insomnia, in order that I might
be protected, especially during my vacations. He suffered over separations, and dreaded them, telling me he wanted me not to enjoy
my time away from him. It was very noticeable that, although this
rise in the levels of contact with his true self, and aggression, was
exactly accompanied by better sleep on less medication, he never
acknowledged the part that analysis (thus, I) had played in bringing about the improvement.

For a long time I could not decide whether this inability to acknowledge me was due to splitting, and what Bion has called attacks on linking, or whether it was his envious meanness. On reflection now, I would say it was undoubtedly both. Unless his own
narcissism was being regularly fed by a relationship (other than with
me, of course), he could be so hurtfully grudging that I realized it
was a form of sadism; an example of him being "permitted" to be
generous was during a glamorous relationship he had for a couple
of years with a famous American star of stage and screen, who genuinely seemed to have fallen heavily for him; he could not speak highly
enough of all her near-perfect attributes. He did, by the way, have
a surprising number of sexual affairs in his life, and a proportion
of the women stayed loyal to him and enabled him to develop the
nearest he could come to friendship. I say "surprising" because to
me he seemed peculiarly unattractive in all sorts of ways, including

sexually; he was quite good-looking but he grimaced, and groaned, and cracked his knuckles much of the time. Also, as with many deeply neurotic people, his skin was grayish, and very slightly damp (I could see a sort of glisten on it) and I well recall the wettish flabby handshake when I first met him. He was what the Buddhists would call *akusala*, "unwholesome"! And, as I indicated right at the beginning, he smelled. This continued, strong and offensive, until I could bring myself to begin to interpret it as part of his message to me and the world; I pointed out that it was not only actively aggressive but also it said: "I am uncared for." The smell abated somewhat, but I never developed warmth toward him, and, as I discussed in several papers in my first book, *Slouching Towards Bethlehem* (1992), the special kind of love that is such a regular feature of our particular long, deep intimacy with most of our patients; and I do not think this absence was simply due to him not being "my type," or anything banal of that nature. I believe it said something about a crippling deficiency in his mother's early preverbal relationship to him, and to his true self, and projectively I became the cold and critical, unloving, "bad" mother. Insofar as this was countertransference, which I liked to believe at least some of it was, it was quite a difficult one to handle.

Finally, there was another feature of the analysis that I gradually realized was capable of releasing him from his mind's torment, which kept him awake while it tried to force him to sleep. This was a certain sort of discussion about suicide. He had, several times in his life, the first at age 14, come closer than do most people to realizing recurring fantasies of suicide. I remember being considerably helped by the writings of Winnicott and of Guntrip when I was working with John. He was deeply capable of what Winnicott called the "fear of annihilation," and yet he could, paradoxically, think about creating his own annihilation, largely because to control himself and his mind and its fears was a dominant wish with him. I did not consider that he had already brought about his own inner psychic death long ago, as Guntrip describes in some of the most deadly, empty, schizoid patients: John had plenty of real anxieties, and hidden true feelings. But he was afraid of the strength of these.

Where I felt Guntrip had accurately divined part of John's existential anguish was in what he called the "tragic self-contradictoriness in the problem of schizoid suicide." He adds: "The longing to die represents the schizoid need to withdraw the ego from a world that is too much for it to cope with. All available energy goes into a quiet but tenacious determination to fade into oblivion by means of gas, hypnotic pills or drowning." (Guntrip 1968, pp. 81–82). On each occasion—five in all—John had been what he called "saved" (which was his more rational ego speaking) by becoming hypomanic. It was quite clear from his description of the emotional state that had supervened to deflect him that it was certainly hypomania. Eventually there was one occurrence during the analysis, the only occasion when I had become seriously concerned about him, and allowed him to ring me through a weekend; it was precipitated by a firm and quite unexpected rejection from the glamorous film star. I welcomed the hypomania then as much as he did, and of course it enabled him to become very aggressive toward me, which was most valuable, and also to be truly witty for a change. He regarded himself as a sophisticated wit, and was often pained and angry when I did not respond to his rather labored, and, to me, unfunny humor. I would have shown it if I had appreciated it, although as I was quite near the beginning of my career as an analyst, I doubt whether I would have laughed in the uninhibited way that I find so easy at this end of my professional life.

The sort of discussion that initiated sleep rather than insomnia was one in which he would find that a truer self became accessible, as he hesitantly tried to explore the inner meanings of the dangerously real attraction that suicide held for him. It seemed that there *was*, alongside what I said earlier, a simple, genuinely felt equation between death and sleep. He could enter a near-delusional state in which he had but to will the end and provide the means and he would, after all, be able to induce peaceful sleep by this act of will (mind). When he swung up into the rescuing hypomanic state, he would accuse himself violently of "lunatic bloody nonsense." If we did not reach the necessary level of deep and concentrated attention in our talk about it, he would feel shame and fear about various aspects of what he thought; he feared being accused of "boasting," for a start. He *was* a boastful man, and he knew it, and it caused him considerable anguish. Then he feared being mocked and humiliated instead of being understood; he feared being told he "didn't mean it," that his fantasies were shallow and unreal, and, with the part of him in which this was also true, he felt ashamed. These scornful and humiliating attacks all derived from a powerful internal figure that bore considerable resemblance to, and was indeed based on, the true selves of his parents in their cold and bored relationship to him. (Ultimately, of course, their derisive belittling served to protect *them* from the narcissistic attack on them represented by his suicidal thoughts.) But he could eventually get deeper inside himself and, as it were, bypass this figure, and then we could, through our close empathic attention, relieve him of his torment and insomnia. Insofar as he had also experienced a good side to his mother, which belonged rather to his middle childhood than to his infancy, he had reinforced it with wishful ideas, and it was with this figure that he sought the prototypical reconciliation that he sometimes tried to effect with me. Above all, in death he longed for such a reunion, and in his nearest approaches to suicide believed that he would find it, and with it, rest and peace and bliss.

The analysis of John and his mind proceeded thus for six years, and then we began to think about stopping, for in many ways he had made real improvements, not least in somewhat better sleep and in the experiencing of a more natural and unforced access to true self elements. He expressed himself as "about as satisfied as I'm ever likely to be, and you know what a critical bugger I am." Of course, we could have done more—one often feels that, and I believe it is right that one should. But I felt it more strongly with him than with many patients. At least I could be aware that in feeling inclined to stop he was not necessarily striving to please me, which had frequently been one of his modes of being in the analysis. He thoroughly understood by then the entrapping double bind of wanting to be better because the other person wanted and needed it (which

brought huge resistance into his own drive to health). He had tried
to ensure that my narcissism did not receive much gratification from
any of the distinct improvements he knew about. He still called the
check he gave me each month "your unearned income"! His leaving was markedly eased by our agreed decision that he should have
some group analysis; we had discussed this at length, and eventually, with his agreement, I had referred him to a friend of mine,
the director of the Group Analytic Practice, who had offered him a
place in the group he ran for "mature people with social difficulties." John left analysis in mid-1973.

Four years later, he wrote me a brief note, enclosing a small check
for a charity I was connected with, saying simply that he had seen
that they were mounting an appeal and he would like to contrib-
ute. I wrote a note to thank him; I remember that I thought about
the appeal, to *him*, of an "appeal" for a kind of help. Five days later,
I received a letter from a friend and colleague of his at the university, who said that I might not have heard that he had died; what
she could not know was that it was on the day after he sent the
check, and the anniversary of the date he had left analysis. She
added: "Apparently it was his own decision." So his mind, the spoiler
of his life, won in the end; it seemed he had not sufficiently internalized my therapeutic value to him in my absence. He must have
felt very confident that I would come to know of his death and the
date on which he arranged it, for I imagine the date was entirely
and consciously a last attacking signal to me. And indeed, alongside the letter, the next day there was a notice in *The Times*, which
he knew I read. It was not just a death announcement; it was a
paragraph about him and his work (he had written two books on
philosophical subjects). He must have known that an obituary was
prepared, as the subjects of them are consulted when they are written. I was sorry that he was not there to see it in print; it is a true
mark of specialness and esteem to get an obituary in *The Times* and
his narcissism would have relished it. He left no notes for anyone,
and knowing the temptation that writing a note would have offered
to his verbosity and his histrionic talent, I admired the dignity and
forbearance of his silent departure.

REFERENCES

Coltart, N. (1992). *Slouching Towards Bethlehem*. London; Free Association.

Freud, S. (1916). Some character-types met with in psychoanalytic work: those wrecked by success. *Standard Edition:* 316–331.

Guntrip, H. (1968). *Schizoid Phenomena, Object Relations and the Self*. London: Hogarth.

Kohut, H. (1990). *The Search for the Self*, ed. A. Goldberg. New York: International Universities Press.

Lacan, J. (1977). *Ecrits: a Selection*, trans. A. Sheridan. London and New York: Tavistock/Norton.

Winnicott, D. W. (1968). *The Maturational Processes and the Facilitating Environment*. London: Hogarth.

3

The Development of Mind-as-Object

Harold Stewart

It has been noted that some patients' mental functioning, particularly their pride in intellectual powers and abilities, prevents them from recognizing their markedly impaired ability to feel emotions and to sense bodily activities. Their minds are not at one with their bodies and this discrepancy has usually been present since childhood. Characteristically, they have been unwilling to notice any deficiencies in themselves since they tend to have an exaggerated and inflated sense of their superiority over others, together with an intense rivalry with, and envy of, the capacities of others. As adults, they tend to come to treatment when circumstances make them aware of the emptiness of their lives in spite of their achievements and their inability to form satisfactory relationships with others. Their diagnoses are usually narcissistic or borderline personality.

Freud suggested in *The Disposition to Obsessional Neurosis* (1913) that "the possibility that a chronological outstripping of libidinal development by ego development should be included in the disposition to obsessional neurosis" (p. 325). This is clearly a feature not only of obsessional neurosis but also of the narcissistic and borderline personality disorders. He further remarked that "we shall be inclined to regard some degree of this precocity of ego development as typical of human nature and to derive the capacity for the origin

of morality from the fact that in the order of development hate is
the precursor of love." Although Freud wrote that this precocity
was typical of human nature, he nevertheless linked it with the idea
of hate being the precursor of love. This suggests he had an inkling
of the importance of hate in ego-precocity, which was to be an
important dynamic in later developments in the clinical study of
such patients, where the influence of hate and its derivatives can
be seen. This dynamic leads us to consider carefully the role of hate
in the development of mind-as-object.

Following Freud, Ferenczi, particularly in his paper "Confusion
of Tongues Between Adults and the Child" (1933), described the
effect of the misuse of children by adults. "The weak and undevel-
oped personality reacts to sudden unpleasure not by defence, but
by anxiety-ridden identifications and by introjection of the menacing
person or aggressor" (p. 163). At the same time, there is a "traumatic
progression, a precocious maturity" in which the child "changes
into psychiatrist and, in order to become one and to defend himself against dangers coming from people without self-control, he must
know how to identify himself completely with them" (p.165). The
child splits his ego and becomes a "wise child," relying on his precociously matured intellectual abilities to deal with the environmental hazards at the expense of his emotional and bodily experiences
and development.

In "Mind and Its Relation to the Psyche-Soma" (1949) Winnicott
developed this theme of the mind–body split particularly in the
child's earliest experiences of its mothering.

> One might ask what happens if the strain that is put on mental
> functioning organized in defence against a tantalizing early envi-
> ronment is greater and greater? One would expect confusional
> states. . . . As a more common result of the lesser degrees of tanta-
> lizing infant care in the earliest stages we find mental functioning
> becomes a thing in itself, practically replacing the good mother and
> making her unnecessary. Clinically this can go along with depen-
> dence on the actual mother and a false personal growth on a com-
> pliant basis. [p. 246]

CASE STUDY

The psychopathology and familial development of the type of patient we are discussing are seen in a married woman, advanced in her profession, who, at the time of this session, had been in analysis for several years.

P: I feel rather mad, my thoughts don't join up with the things I do and I'm afraid there's something wrong with my mind. I feel cold even though I'm warmly dressed and I feel all alone like the baby who's been left in the pram between feeds.

A: You feel I've just been cold to you between sessions leaving you alone to face your confused thoughts and possible madness by yourself.

P: Yes. You don't care about me at all . . . (and she makes other similar comments about my lack of caring and I respond by allowing myself to be seen as responsible for her painful state).

P: Now I feel better with your interpretations.

A: How do you mean?

P: You don't tell me it's all my fault but show understanding for the way I feel and I like that. But I don't know if you're just seducing me by talking to me like that and not really meaning it at all. Are you just trying to trick me by it? Perhaps I've been saying these things in order to get you to interpret like that in a sympathetic manner and so I'm really seducing you to trick you. I get so confused.

A: You feel that if you do get something from me that pleases you, it's not genuine on my part or it's been obtained by non-genuine means by you.

P: That's right and I always feel the same thing with my mother. (Her mother has been described consistently as a domineering and depressed woman and her father as a rather inadequate, obsessional man.)

In the next session, which started with a long silence, she then said that she liked the fact that I'd spoken a lot yesterday as she liked listening to the sound of my voice and it was like being in a warm bath. She also said that she knew that when she had said this on previous occasions, I had interpreted that she preferred listening to the sound of my voice rather than the meaning of what I had actually said, so she knew that she was avoiding thinking about any meaning to yesterday's session.

At the beginning of her analysis, this patient had used her mind in a different way. She handled the analytic discourse constructively, listening to my interpretations and building on them. But it gradually became apparent that this was based on false pretenses. These intellectual, analytical constructions based on our discourse were being used not in the service of true genuine insight and meaning but as a defensive intellectual process, both to comply with what she thought I wanted and to obsure her feelings of inner emptiness. This void was partly created to hide states of inner confusion and chaos, and suicidal thoughts. Such states are usually associated with early deficiencies of parenting by typically dominating, depressed mothers and inadequate fathers.

This patient's clinical material illustrates the states of mind that have appeared since the intellectualizing phase has been largely given up during the course of the analysis. She is confused, feels angry, and is suspicious of herself and of the analyst, particularly when she feels understood by him. Her defense against this paranoid-schizoid state of mind is to cease hearing the contents of her thoughts and my interpretations and instead concentrate on the warmth in my voice to nullify her suspicions of my seductive trickiness. In this way she is also demonstrating the destruction of the new meanings and insight that I have given her during the analysis, a clear indication of her extreme envy of my capacities as an analyst to understand minds in ways that she had not first thought of herself. This has long been a source of severe humiliation to her as a mind-as-object. The destruction of meaning has also effected a further emphasis of the body–mind split, because with her simple warm-bath feeling, she avoids any painful bodily sensations that would be associated with feeling separate from the analyst. These states of destructive envy and dread of separation are associated with severe early deficiency states related to the primary objects in the environment.

The patient, in her opening comments, had been "afraid that there's something wrong with my mind." Previously she had believed that she had a first-class mind, all-knowing, and capable of precise logical thinking, but it gradually became evident, to her distress, that she didn't know as much as she thought she did, that her ideas were rather fixed, and her reasoning sometimes faulty and illogical. One aspect of my technique with her in these early phases was to try to understand how her mind did work in its thinking processes; this was done by occasionally questioning her illogicalities and certainties without giving my opinion on them and noting her responses to these minor confrontations. Whenever she experienced her mind as not being the perfect instrument she thought it was, she became affronted by my questioning and mocked me in a superior fashion. I might then interpret her response as her intense dislike of being questioned by someone she felt was her intellectual inferior. To acknowledge any intellectual defects made her feel inferior, worthless, and humiliated, and so for her to eventually experience something wrong with her mind was a humiliating defeat and a dreadful setback in treatment. Insofar as the supposed superiority of her mind had been based on the clarity achieved by splitting, denial, and omniscience, the mind-as-object was now collapsing in its importance to her, leaving her with the underlying confusion and paranoid suspicions. She felt this as a deterioration while also gradually realizing that it was a positive development in the search for the childhood states of mental functioning, with all its confusions and uncertainties, in relationship to her parental objects. It is important to maintain this clinically regressed state by having frequent sessions, because if the time between sessions is too long, the intellectualizing processes will rapidly reassert themselves to avoid the painful emotional states inherent in the clinical situation. The various theories of the development of mind-as-object shortly to be described all stress the defensive use of this state against such painful emotional states as those seen in the clinical situation.

Let us examine further Winnicott's views of the mind-as-object. As a result of the excessive impingements on the infant from the mother or her substitute, the infant becomes compliant with the mother's needs, demands, and emotional states, and thus will not attack the mother either aggressively or destructively in the way a normal infant would with a good-enough mother. Winnicott postulated in "The Use of an Object" (1969) that the way that the infant achieves objective, real separation from the mother is to subject her to aggressive and destructive attacks. When these attacks are inhibited by compliance, the infant will not separate but remain attached both internally and externally to the mother, who is perceived as a subjective object. At the same time, the infant identifies with the mother's feelings and states of mind, with her omnipotence and narcissism. In this way, the infant attempts constantly to understand and know the mother and then to please her by fitting in with what the infant thinks the mother wants. This will also occur on a reparative basis, with the infant acting, as Ferenczi suggested, as the mother's psychiatrist. In this way, the mind is an object not only in the sense that it is separated prematurely from the psyche-soma, but also in the sense that it is mother's mind and not the infant's. The mind will tend to think in terms of splitting, of extremes of good and bad, and in black-and-white terms: but behind this so-called clarity will be confusion and chaos. This confusion will consist both of the infant's confusional state behind the compliance and splitting and of the mother's confusional state behind her own omnipotence and narcissism. These features can regularly be found in the analysis of these types of patients.

> In the early years of her analysis, the patient had believed her mother to be a wonderful loving woman, intelligent, and a brilliant conversationalist. The mother had frequent depressive states, which were blamed on the exigencies of the mother's early years, and during these states, the patient and her father had tiptoed around the mother. Often while speaking of her mother, the patient talked of her loneliness and excessive docility as a child in the face of her mother's violent tempers, and it was only later in the analysis that she saw that the mother dominated and controlled the family. She had had to fit in from an early age and identify almost completely with the mother to avoid both the frightening tempers and being excluded by a depressed withdrawal. She felt she had been tricked and seduced into being good, hard-working, and intelligent and didn't know whether any of her achievements were her own or her mother's.

She came to hate her mother with a fierce intensity; "I don't know if I'm me or my mother." This hatred of the mother was mirrored in the transference by her destructive attacks on the analyst, one factor being her envy of his mind, which she gradually realized was not crippled like her own. The analyst's survival of these repeated attacks is one of the factors that Winnicott postulates is essential for the patient's perception of the analyst (and internalized parent) as a subjective object to change to the perception of the analyst as a real, objective, and separate object. The analyst is performing the paternal function of coming between mother and child as a symbiotic duo and helping in their separation, an important function for the establishment in the infant and patient of their own mind–body integration.

Because such mothers tend to have married inadequate or compliant husbands, the fathers will not have the necessary aggressive virility to come between infant and mother and effect the separation in the infant–mother duo and to provide a paternal model for the infant. This function will be one of the tasks for the analyst to effect during the course of the therapy. In this form of family configuration, the child has had to accommodate herself to the mother's emotional and mental state by identification in order to attempt to maintain the mother's equilibrium. The father's absence makes him unable to be of much use to the mother in this respect, and even when he is with the family his own emotional inadequacies and conflictual states with the mother only aggravate the situation. The child is in the position of having to try to take the father's place to make up for his inadequacies, which has the effect of increasing the child's feelings of omnipotence over not only the mother but the father, too; the father is often held in contempt by both mother and child. The other side of the coin is the hatred that the child feels for being placed in this position, for not being held and supported as a child but rather having to be the parent to the parents. Under these circumstances, the child's mind is forced to identify with and become the parents' mind in order to learn how they function. As the child's feeling states, particularly of hatred, loss, despair, and confusion, thus must be denied, the mind-as-object state takes over as the child's most valuable possession, even though it is erected on a false-mind basis. It is false because it is based not on the healthy, slow integration of one's own mind with that of one's parents in a healthy child–parent configuration, but rather on the pathological modes already described.

Michael Balint's theories are relevant to this consideration of mind-as-object. Starting from his concept of primary object-love, in which the biological basis is the mutual interdependence of mother and infant together with a harmonious mix of subject and object, firm, discrete objects emerge as a result of the inevitable frustrations and separations between infant and mother. If considerable discrepancies arise at this stage between the biopsychological needs of the infant and the material and psychological care of the maternal figure, a basic fault, a structural deficiency, will develop in the mind of the infant. From this basic fault, two character types may develop, each in its way similar to Winnicott's false-self state. The first type is the ocnophile, which experiences objects as safe and friendly but the space between objects as hostile and threatening; the second is the philobat, where the converse is the case—the space between objects is experienced as safe and friendly but the objects are potentially threatening. Usually there is a mixture of these types, and it is from this mixture that the mind-as-object phenomenon will emerge (Balint 1959).

Balint suggested that a special characteristic of philobatic type is a very high development of ego skills, which enables the philobat to maintain its independence from its potentially dangerous objects. These ego skills can be of different functions in different people, and I would suggest that precocious overdevelopment of intellectual skills and mental functioning in the mind-as-object patient is an example of philobatic functioning. The states of compliance and suspiciousness that are found in these patients arise from the mixture of philobatic and ocnophilic states, with the ocnophilic compliance arising from its relationship to a potentially dangerous object of which one is suspicious. Balint (1959) speaks of the almost magical properties of the philobat's experience of his skills; Winnicott (1949) also refers to "the almost magical healing properties of these patients because of their extreme capacity to make active adaptations to primitive needs" (p. 247). The patient described in the case study here was very much the intellectual philobat in the early years of the analysis, while at the same time showing the ocnophilic, clinging, compliant characteristics.

Wilfred Bion's (1962) theory of thinking is a different theory of the mind from that of Freud's. Bion starts with the assumption that thinking is dependent on two mental developments: the development of thoughts, and the development of an apparatus to cope with them, which he calls "thinking." The apparatus develops to cope with the pressure of thoughts, as opposed to the more usual idea that thoughts are the product of thinking. He classified thoughts into preconceptions, conceptions, and concepts. A *preconception* corresponds to the infant's inborn disposition to the expectation of a breast; if this preconception is brought into contact with what Bion calls the realization of the experience of a satisfying breast, this mental outcome of preconception and its realization is called a *conception*. If however, this preconception is brought into contact with the realization of the experience of an absent breast, or as Bion calls it, a no-breast available for satisfaction, the mental outcome will be dependent on the capacity of the infant for tolerance of the frustration inherent in this no-breast experience. If the capacity for the tolerance of frustration is sufficient, which is based on previous conceptions of the experience of satisfaction, then this experience of the no-breast inside becomes a *concept*, a thought, and an apparatus for thinking the thought develops, i.e., a rudimentary mind. If, however, this capacity for tolerance is insufficient, then processes of modification or evasion become necessary.

Bion further introduced ideas known as alpha function and beta elements. The essential feature of *alpha function* is the process of generating meaning out of new sensory data, which is linked with the capacity to tolerate frustrations of the sensory data of the no-breast experience for the production of thoughts. If this capacity for tolerance is inadequate, alpha functioning fails, with the result that particles of undigested sensory data, or *beta elements*, accumulate in the psyche and are dealt with by evacuation, a form of evasion. The development of the capacity for alpha functioning in the infant depends on the capacity of the mother to contain and manage the infant's projective identifications of unwanted feelings, such as the fear of dying. These are beta elements that are being evacuated into the mother, who will then act on them with her own alpha functioning to make them into a more manageable form for the infant to be able to receive them back through reintrojection. In this way the mother enables the infant to develop his own capacity for alpha functioning both directly and by identification with the mother.

However, and here we come to the mind-as-object theme, if the mother's ability to tolerate and contain these projections of the infant is defective, the development of the infant's alpha functioning will also be defective to varying degrees. Bion suggests that if the maternal intolerance is not too great, omniscience and omnipotence will arise as a substitute for the mating of the preconception or conception with the negative realization. In addition to this, he postulates a precocious development of consciousness, which he uses in Freud's terms to mean a "sense organ for the perception of psychic qualities" (1900, Chapter 7). The idea of psychic qualities refers to the meaning and significance of things. Since there is a deficiency of alpha functioning, this sense organ will be deficient in its perception of sense data of the self, particularly those arising from bodily and emotional sources. In this way there arises the mental state of a person relatively dominated by omnipotence and omniscience together with a deficiency of appreciation of body and emotional self-states. This is the state of mind-as-object.

To return to the case study, we can see that in the session described an interactive dialogue is going on and that an analytic type of understanding is being shown by both the analyst and the patient. The patient's mind is still being used in a defensive manner over the issues of seduction and trickery and over the avoidance of thinking about the meaning of my statements, but nevertheless the expression of doubts and feeling states are now present in the analysis. This defensive use of the mind seems to me to be of a different order from the mind-as-object state, where omnipotence, omniscience, projective identification, denial, splitting, contempt, and the relative absence of feelings are the prevailing defensive mechanisms. The patient is becoming more integrated and the manic defenses of the mind-as-object state are lessening and becoming more depressive in nature. This mind-as-object state can be regarded as a form of a pathological defensive organization (Steiner 1987).

CASE STUDY

The most extreme example that I have encountered is that of a patient with an encapsulated psychosis whose experience of the analytic situation was that my room did not exist, nor did he and I; the only thing that existed was something called his mind, described as a bowl into which my voice passed, and it was located in a boundless void. He came to me because he believed he had changed into the woman who had just recently deserted him and he felt suicidal. He felt he contained no love, only hate and some pity. I soon discovered he believed he was God, all-wise and all-powerful. He had a black, mordant sense of humor, particularly when I empathized with his withering contempt for others, including his analyst, and for their human failings and vulnerabilities; in this black humor he resembled the patient described by Bollas (Chapter 5). After very many years of therapy he now knows that he and I are in the room speaking to each other and that he is not God, but he is not yet completely sure whether there is any reality outside of his mind. Apart from endless time and patience, the technique I found to be most useful was not one of interpretations, transference or otherwise, since they were meaningless to him, but rather one of accepting and analyzing his omnipotence and omniscience by querying his logic and conclusions in terms of his own statements to me. I naturally did not introduce reality to him or put forward my views on anything but got him to question his own. At the same time I needed to empathize with whoever or whatever he believed himself to be at different phases of the analysis, such as God, or a tyrant king, or an ancient stone rock. Only in this way could my queries or observations on what he might be feeling make any sense to him, although it was very tricky to know what an inanimate ancient stone might be thinking or experiencing. What I was trying to do was to help him to examine all his conceptions and preconceptions so that the small area of sanity of mind could understand gradually his insanity. Every piece of insight was accompanied by humiliation and shame as his omnipotent facade developed cracks. His mind-as-object was not experienced as his own, particularly as he had no self, but gradually it became less split-off and its omnipotence and omniscience were reduced as some of his split-off projective identifications of mind and self started to return. As for his family, his mother was a dominant and intelligent woman who could not bear physical contact with her children, his father was ineffectual but a family tyrant, and a sibling was schizophrenic. This does seem a telling pattern for mind-as-object states.

In conclusion, the principal common factor, following Ferenczi, of the three theories mentioned in the development of this state is the paramount importance of the external environment, particularly of the primary maternal figure. Winnicott speaks of the excessive impingement that occurs when this maternal functioning is not good enough in its holding function; Balint speaks of the discrepancy that arises between the biopsychological needs of the infant and the quality of maternal caregiving; and Bion speaks of the deficiency of the containing function and provision of alpha functioning by the maternal figure. With these deficiencies, normal healthy development of psyche-soma functioning cannot occur and the pathological mind-as-object state arises in its place.

REFERENCES

Balint, M. (1959). Philobatism and ocnophilia. In *Thrills and Regressions*. London: Hogarth.

Bion, W. R. (1962). A theory of thinking. *International Journal of Psycho-Analysis* 43:306–310.

Ferenczi, S. (1933). Confusion of tongues between adults and the child. In *Final Contributions to the Problems and Methods of Psychoanalysis*, ed. M. Balint. London: Hogarth.

Freud, S. (1900). The interpretation of dreams. *Standard Edition* 5:615.

—— (1913). The disposition to obsessional neurosis. *Standard Edition* 12:325.

Steiner, J. (1987). The interplay between pathological organizations and the paranoid-schizoid and depressive positions. *International Journal of Psycho-Analysis* 68:69–80.

Winnicott, D. W. (1949). Mind and its relation to the psyche-soma. In *Collected Papers: Through Paediatrics to Psychoanalysis.* London: Tavistock, 1958.

—— (1969). The use of an object. *International Journal of Psycho-Analysis* 50:711–716.

4

"Understanding Too Much" The Treatment of a Precocious Young Boy

Edward G. Corrigan
Pearl-Ellen Gordon[1]

UNDERSTANDING TOO MUCH

If we take the case of a baby whose mother's failure to adapt is too rapid, we can find that the baby survives by means of the mind. . . . If the baby has a good mental apparatus this thinking becomes a substitute for maternal care and adaptation. The baby "mothers" himself by means of understanding, understanding too much. [Winnicott 1965, p. 156]

Simon, a few days before his third birthday, greets me in a friendly and eager manner. Entering the office with his mother behind him, he glances at the toys with apparent delight, but almost immediately asks for the markers. Quickly, he and his mother settle into a drawing and role playing game that in its compulsive repetition has become an all-too-familiar scenario in his family. Disney's *The Little Mermaid* has captured Simon's imagination; he assigns the role of

---

1. This chapter is a collaborative effort of the authors who discussed Simon's ongoing treatment. Dr. Corrigan was the therapist.

Ariel, the little mermaid, to his mother while he alternates between the roles of King Triton, Ariel's worried and angry father, and Ursula, the greedy sea-witch. He has his mother draw lines on a page of paper that represent Ariel's toys, and with his trident his yellow marker, he angrily crosses them out. Simon looks at his mother and threatens her, "Ariel, I am going to break your toys!" His mother replies, "Oh no, Daddy, don't break my toys, please don't." The game repeats itself until Simon requests "copies," and his mother produces Xeroxed copies from *The Little Mermaid* coloring book.

Simon seems eager now to tell me about the drama of *The Little Mermaid* and with his mother interpreting his somewhat difficult to capture articulations, he describes a story of a greedy witch and an enraged and possessive king who is terribly threatened by his daughter's wish to leave him. In retaliation he breaks her toys with a frightening bolt of fire magically struck from his trident. (The toys represent the artifacts that she has collected from the human world.) Again and again, with his yellow marker serving as his fiery trident, Simon threatens Ariel, "I am going to break your toys!" I ask the little king, "Why are you so angry at Ariel?" Simon repeats a line from the story—King Triton's justification for his angry destruction of Ariel's treasured human objects. "Human beings are dangerous," Simon tells me. He asks for water for the water paints, and he asks me which brush is fine or thick. Now with his paint brush, he continues to break Ariel's toys, occasionally threatening his mother or myself directly with his trident. Intently engaged in his task, his eyes glued to the paper before him, and in a faraway voice, Simon asks a stunning, almost rhetorical question: "How are we to understand all of this?" His mother and I are both astonished and we look at him in disbelief. Without looking up from his work, Simon repeats his question, "How are we to understand all of this?"

In Chapter 1 we presented a theoretical framework upon which we based our observations that certain patients, in order to manage overwhelming anxieties, seemed to have turned, omnipotently, to their mind—establishing it as their most reliable object. In this chapter, we present details from the first three years of Simon's therapy. We believe Simon's unfolding case material provides a special opportunity to study key early phenomena in the formation of the mind as an object.

THE FIRST PHASE OF TREATMENT

Simon's parents, Mr. and Mrs. Smith, were referred when Simon was two. They had become increasingly concerned about their son's repeated temper tantrums, which, at their worst, would last nearly three hours and often seemed to erupt with no apparent cause. Simon was inconsolable at these times. He would bang his head on the floor, turn over furniture, thrash about helplessly, and would finally only be relieved by exhaustion.

Although I had observed Simon in a play setting, during the first year of contact with the family, I worked with Simon's parents, seeing them as a couple as well as individually. These sessions constituted the first stage in what has amounted to three phases of treatment. In the second phase, I saw Simon and his mother in twice a week conjoint sessions, while continuing to meet regularly with his parents both individually and as a couple. In the third (ongoing) phase, Simon is being seen individually, three times a week, at first, and then, two times a week.

Simon's father pointed out that with Simon there was no middle ground. He was either a fiercely stubborn, raging, impossible child or a charming, engaging, brilliant companion. His parents described Simon as possessing an astonishing memory and vocabulary. He knew his letters, his numbers, and his colors and shapes. He talked in sentences early and had what his parents described as advanced communication skills. In a delightful manner, he sought the approval of adults, although he avoided altogether the company of his peers. He had a bright sense of humor, and he tried to make his parents laugh by asking them to remember funny events. Noticing his father's frustration about something, Simon teased, "Daddy, you can't do everything you want to do!"

While his parents were disappointed that Simon would never allow them to hold him, comfort him, or cuddle with him—Simon would always squirm and wiggle away—they actively promoted his independence and self-management. They were proud of the fact that Simon would "never cry for us—never want us." They would never allow him to come into their bedroom, either for play and fun, or when distressed in the middle of the night. Thus, in many ways, Mr. and Mrs. Smith had encouraged and applauded Simon's self-sufficient, precocious behavior. Looking to Simon to fulfill various unrealized longings within themselves, they described his birth as like that of the Dalai Lama—such was their reverence.

Their idealization of Simon had a variety of consequences for the family's organizational patterns. In particular, it undermined their authority. They were loath to establish boundaries and set limits. Roles had been reversed, and Simon had come to rule his parents. As Mr. Smith confessed, they were the "adoring servants, he the Gestapo parent."

During the first few months of periodic consultations, a picture emerged of a family caught up in interlocking webs of debilitating unconscious conflicts unable to make use of their own considerable resources. Indeed, there were "ghosts in the nursery" (Fraiberg 1980), and Simon, perhaps an intellectually gifted child, appeared, to us, to be attempting to cope with his anxiety by the creation of a precocious defense. Mrs. Smith had become significantly depressed, agitated, and withdrawn during Simon's first year of life. It was clear that Simon's experience of his mother's unavailability, coupled with various of his father's problems in parenting, had created a painful, angry schism, in particular between Simon and his mother, as well as a precarious void in Simon's evolving sense of self. We understood Simon's developing precocity, in part, as a very sensitive infant's attempt to manage what we imagined as states of acute stress that were generated as his mother and father's moments of anxiety, anger, competition, and withdrawal impinged upon him. His fierce and prolonged tantrums expressed his inner torment. At first, Simon had turned to his father, who later confessed that he had competed with his wife, wanting to be the better parent. Now Simon favored his father and his baby-sitter over his mother. "Daddy hold . . . only Daddy . . . Mommy out" were his angry commands. And he used his favoritism of his father vindictively to get even with his mother. In the end, Simon made his point, and it was his mother who initiated the consultation.

On the basis of the information that we had collected over the first months of consultation, I discussed with the family what we saw as the most pressing issue facing them—the serious breakdown in the relationship between Simon and his mother. Aware of the complexity of the situation and recognizing the time needed to sort out the issues, we also heard the urgency of Simon's enraged communication. As a first step, I encouraged Mrs. Smith to reorganize her part-time work schedule so that she and Simon could spend more continuous time together, and also suggested regressive kinds of play such as finger painting, previously an altogether too messy activity for Simon (See James 1960). While cognizant of Mrs. Smith's anxiety, we also appreciated her motivation and capacity for insight. Thus, we hoped that this kind of play along with Mrs. Smith's increased availability would begin to counter the need for Simon's reliance on premature ego functioning, while, in time, her increased psychic availability might help give Simon a restorative experience of dependency.

This initial intervention seemed to succeed, at least, at first. Simon's tantrums did subside as he and his mother hesitantly began to find more pleasure in each other. However, seven months into this phase of the treatment, the family moved to a new house, and after a brief, relaxed period of settling-in, Mrs. Smith resumed her part-time work schedule, and Simon's rage erupted with even greater intensity, demanding eventually a different mode of intervention.

However, before we describe the second phase of treatment, the work with Simon and his mother, let us look more closely at Simon, and his evolving precocious personality organization.

SIMON

To begin with, Simon had always been preoccupied with highly repetitive activities; he would, for example, stack cards or empty and replace kitchen cabinets for hours. But after the family moved, Simon discovered "markering," and his father had reproduced thousands of Xeroxed copies from *The Little Mermaid* coloring book that Simon might insistently "marker" for up to six or eight hours a day. Simon could not sustain any other activity in which his potential gifts for play could be set in motion. He easily became bored and angry and complained that there was nothing to do. Demanding his parent's constant attention, he, nevertheless, could not participate in extended, reciprocal interaction. For Simon, it appeared, that activities that involved an acceptance of change, difference, and separateness were painfully difficult.

In addition, imitation seemed to be an important mode of organization. Simon would become like the characters he read about or saw on video, insisting he be addressed in character, or he would imitate children he met on the playground. His daily conversation was replete with lines he would spontaneously recite from videos or books. To some extent, this had a charming and funny effect, but it made one uneasy, as if Simon's conversation were not emanating from within him, not generated by object relationship, but from some surface imitation meant to entertain his parents and enliven himself.

Related to this kind of phenomenon was Simon's use of language, which seemed to serve a number of purposes other than communication. For example, in one session Simon began to make a painting with huge globs of red paint. He covered the red over with blue, then black, creating a purple color. This was a vivid painting and he seemed frightened. Simon pointed at the purple color and he happily told me that the new color was "plum." It was suddenly hard to resist the charm of this moment, indeed such moments were often celebrated by the family; but if we think that Simon was trying to express the intensity of his feelings with his bold painting, then we can see that his use of words deflected or dispersed emotional experience.

Along similar lines, when Simon asks in the first session, "How are we to understand all of this?" we are at first startled by the apparent sophistication of this 3-year-old. But Simon is obviously imitating or incorporating the adults' use of language, if not their exact phrasing. Here he has prematurely taken on the adult's role and he attempts to "mother" himself by understanding, but to quote Winnicott, "understanding too much."

While the clever use of language, as well as the quick, nearly seamless imitation of various fictional characters seem to come easily, more difficult for Simon were his attempts to act grown-up and self-sufficient. His father described his son's dilemma: "He tries to act like the big boys. He fails, of course, and then he screams, sucks his thumb—he's pathetic to watch at such times." Mr. Smith continued to describe how enormously angry Simon became when he is reminded by his physical limitations that he is just a baby. "He can't bear to acknowledge what he can't do."

MR. AND MRS. SMITH

To provide a perspective on the forces that had derailed Simon's development, we turn to a discussion of Mr. and Mrs. Smith—first, to his mother and the origins of this intelligent and perceptive woman's difficulties in mothering, and second, to his father and to the complications that this talented man brought to his role as Simon's father.

Responding to significant family difficulties, Mrs. Smith seems to have attempted to raise herself and, like many precocious patients, she strove for self-sufficiency and perfection. "I can't allow anyone to help me because they'll disappoint me. . . . I have to do it by myself."

Her pregnancy was a difficult if not a traumatic one. An episode of premature labor was followed by bed rest for intrauterine growth retardation. Mrs. Smith had an eating disorder and during her pregnancy she was determined not to gain weight. Simon was breast-fed for two weeks before Mrs. Smith's milk dried up. He screamed constantly and settled down only when he started on the bottle, which he drank so furiously that it disturbed observers. During the first year of life, Simon refused his mother's efforts to feed him, rarely finishing any meal. Mrs. Smith worried that Simon was born hungry.

Simon's crying terrified her, and she feared that there was no intervention she could make that would soothe him. She felt overwhelmed by Simon's needs, and if someone else was around, she turned his care over to them. She didn't know what to do with Simon—"I didn't know whether to play with him, read to him, change him, or take him out." Mrs. Smith admitted that she returned to her full-time job when Simon was 8 weeks old to get away from Simon and the fear and anxiety that he generated in her.

It was not until a year and a half after Simon's birth that Mrs. Smith recognized the distance that had been created between herself and her son, and it was after this painful realization that she initiated what turned out to be the first phase of treatment. The second stage of treatment began after the family moved. It was then that I recommended conjoint sessions for Simon and his mother. I also underscored the need for Mrs. Smith to make herself available to Simon on an even more continuous basis than we had established earlier. The new work arrangement that she and her husband arrived at required her to leave her part-time job in favor of free-lance work that would take her out of the home only on Mondays and Fridays. The idea of three continuous days at home with Simon, in the middle of the week, filled her with anxiety and, in a sense, forced a confrontation with herself.

No longer able to get away from Simon, Mrs. Smith, at first, experienced herself as his prisoner and in the long days she now spent with Simon she had to fight the strong impulse to shut the door to be by herself (as her mother had done to her). Whenever Simon cried she felt the same reaction she had when Simon was a newborn—she still feared that there was nothing she could do that would comfort him or transform his rageful state.

Mrs. Smith, motivated, no doubt, by a strong, emerging need to reconnect with her son, and supported by her individual treatment, made significant progress in examining the powerful anxieties that had interfered with her capacity to mother her son. A few weeks after we began the conjoint sessions she began her follow-up session by reflecting upon Simon's first year of life. "I was chronically unwell. I was sick all the time with one thing or another. The minute I ate something I got sick. I thought this weekend . . . this is my mother! How could I have been so sick? . . . I am not sick at all." She went on. "I have been depressed all my life. . . . I've been angry. . . . My mother puts it all outside herself. . . . So have I. I refuse food, I'm obsessive and I'm moody. . . . I attack my husband. It's always there. I never thought I could get to it. I always thought it was just a permanent part of my life." In another session, she discussed her eating problems, which had a bearing on her pregnancy and subsequent feeding difficulties with Simon. "I must have realized long ago," she said, "that it was better to be in a constant state of hunger—I could get used to that—than to take the chance of being satisfied and suffer a disappointment."

Mr. Smith, a resourceful and imaginative father, was guided, as a parent, by a series of absolutes: "Never say no. . . . Never be unavailable. . . . Never seem uninterested." His guidelines, inadvertently, but inevitably, contributed to an unbounded atmosphere that fostered Simon's sense of omnipotence. As Mr. Smith ruefully observed, "Simon is totally under the illusion that he, Simon, is in control." Further, in Mr. Smith's ever-present availability, he offered his son a constant and often lively presence; but unaware and a bit misattuned at times, he exploited Simon's cognitive resources, fostering Simon's precocity with overly sophisticated play and word games.

Mr. Smith's guidelines also reveal his vulnerability. On the one hand, coming from a family who postured specialness, Mr. Smith enjoyed, for a time, the sense of belonging to a group that was superior to others. On the other hand, his actual experience was one of being left out and unheard. His talents were not marked by his parents and this left him struggling with feelings of emptiness and boredom. Further, as the youngest of seven children, his father constantly away on business, separated from his older brothers by a large age difference (eight years), growing up, more or less, with his sisters and mother, Mr. Smith felt more comfortable with women than men.

Mr. and Mrs. Smith both came from families with similar constellations. Both of their mothers had been depressed and hospitalized. Both of their fathers, perhaps at their wives' expense, had excelled. Thus, to the extent that Mrs. Smith struggled with an identification with her mother's helplessness and depression in relation to her father's supercompetence, and, simultaneously, to the extent that Mr. Smith attempted to deny his identification with his sisters and mother and embraced, however anxiously, his father's view of the "Smith" superiority, Mr. and Mrs. Smith were vulnerable to intense and unconscious relivings of their own respective family dynamics. Nearly disabling feelings of competition and envy were generated by these underlying conflicts. Mr. Smith secretly envied the mother's role and competed with his wife. At first, in her panic, Mrs. Smith acceded, relieved to turn Simon's care over to her husband. It was not until much later, after Mrs. Smith gained in her struggle to work out her anxieties and the problems generated by her envious feelings toward Mr. Smith's actual competence, accompanied by Mr. Smith's work on his own envy and competitiveness, that Mr. and Mrs. Smith were able to meaningfully cooperate in their management of Simon.

THE THERAPEUTIC SPACE

The therapist's role in the conjoint treatment phase, as we understood it, was to facilitate a reengagement between Simon and his mother. I tried to create an environment that fostered play and comfort seeking, but also tolerated anger and contained destructiveness. At first, I made only occasional interpretations. Generally, I took a back seat to Simon's and his mother's initiatives with each other. I enjoyed Simon, but I tried not to be seduced by his often startling and bright remarks. Obviously, I did not want to reinforce precocity. I attempted to provide a somewhat timeless, unhurried atmosphere. The sessions began, more or less, when Simon and his mother arrived and ended, anywhere from an hour and a half to an hour and three quarters later. Simon and his mother often spent at least another half hour in the waiting room as she slowly managed their departure with further games and books.

We hoped that this therapeutic setup would work as a holding environment for both Simon and his mother, and as such we hoped it might have the power to facilitate a regression of a particular kind. Perhaps Simon and his mother could both discover a world of primary experiences where they could mutually, unconsciously, process one another, affect one another, and transform one another. Could a baby willing to risk dependency meet up with an alive mother willing to receive him?

THE CONJOINT SESSIONS

Simon, in his enormous struggle to manage his rage, seemed to have found in *The Little Mermaid* role-playing and markering game a containing technique. This compulsive activity, which at times appeared to be nearly autistic, had begun to dominate Simon's time a few months before the beginning of the conjoint sessions, and then it became the main activity over the first few months of therapy.

The game seemed to have multiple meanings. For example, we believe that in the fiery image of "breaking," as in "Ariel, I am going to break your toys," Simon, as King Triton, forcefully and repeatedly expressed the sadistic, destructive forces that had accumulated in him. We also believe that the image of "breaking" conveyed Simon's unconscious knowledge of the agony he had suffered as his lifeline had been broken.

At another level, Ursula, the sea witch who comes in the form of a rather overweight octopus, seemed to stand, on the one hand, for Simon's split-off hunger and greed as well as for his own "meanness," and on the other hand for the bad mother—the internal bad object suffused with his own rage and the external mother perceived as angrily withholding and withdrawing from him. Early, in one session, Simon pointed out how "mean" Ursula is; later in the session, as if he had been pondering his observation, he thoughtfully asked, "Why is she so mean?" For weeks, Simon repeatedly asked his seemingly incomprehensible question.

Ursula, the overweight witch, we should add, was an evocative image for both Simon and his mother. Early in the treatment, I intervened when I realized that Mrs. Smith was overcontrolling Simon's access to food, not only in the session, but at home. With considerable conflict, Mrs. Smith altered her control of Simon's food intake.

King Triton's rage at being abandoned by Ariel was related to Simon's predicament with his mother and represented material close to the surface. Working within the metaphor, I made a simple, initial interpretation, suggesting that King Triton is angry because he did not want Ariel to leave him, he did not want to be alone, and that he is getting even with her by breaking her toys.

Simon eventually expressed his anger more directly. Discontented and restless and telling us he was angry, he began to spill paint and turn over the toys. He threw a block at his mother with unexpected force. His actions were contained by the invention of the throwing game. His mother or I would gather the toys that could be thrown, and Simon, with his back to his mother and facing me, would throw them over his head in the general direction of his mother. The game went on and gradually Simon incorporated into his play one of King Triton's lines—"What do I have to do to get through to you!" After a while, Simon altered the line to make a more personal statement: "The only way I can get through to you is to hurt you!"

There were many sessions when Simon's rage would erupt for no obvious reason, and once a tantrum had begun it was not easily contained. His anger would break right through the facade of a role-playing game—he would not be satisfied playing out the scene between King Triton and Ariel. The "throwing game" did not always work and Simon had to be prevented from throwing objects at his mother or myself. At such times, play would be disrupted for nearly the entire session. He refused help or comfort from his mother and he ignored my interpretative comments. At home, he told his mother he wanted to walk down to the main street so a car could hit him. In other sessions, however, Simon showed his potential for creative, symbolic play. Towards the end of one session, for example, Simon, his mother, and I built a tower upon which Simon placed a little dog. When he knocked over the tower, he pointed out that the dog falls, but he's okay. He designated the dog as the "happy prince" and Simon seemed content. He built a road up to the castle and he placed a bear on the couch and pointed out how the bear "sees everything" from this, the highest point in Simon's imaginary land. Then, to complete the scene he introduced a flying monster who also lives in this land. He is huge and black, and apparently referring to his bad dreams, Simon tells us that the monster "fills the sky with nighttime."

There is some hopefulness in this scenario. The prince on the tower may be an image of his specialness and precocity, but he can fall from this vulnerable position and survive. The road to the castle evokes the possibility of connection. And in the transference, Simon has apparently portrayed me as a benevolent bear—an overseer. Nevertheless, danger lurks in his rage, which fills his dreams.

In a subsequent session, Simon told me that he's likely to be a grouch—he's tired and he hasn't slept very well. We discussed his bad dreams that keep him awake at night and I tell Simon I think I know where the monsters are coming from—that he makes them up out of his anger. Near the end of the session, Simon made a bold, evocative painting of a "happy monster." Why is the monster happy? He is "happy because he has hurt someone."

Perhaps emboldened by his incipient efforts to represent his rage symbolically in this painting and in others, Simon played out his anger at home in an interactive mode with his mother. Expressing his underlying fear of fragmentation, he would pick up an object and ask his mother repetitively, "Will this break? . . . What will happen if I drop this? . . . How many pieces will this break into?" He challenged his mother, earnestly asking her, "What are you going to do if I break this? Will you be so angry that you will break everything?" This kind of testing went on all day and Simon did break a display of dried flowers. He was sent to his room, and when he asked to return his mother warned him against causing any further damage. Simon told his mother, in his wry way, that she didn't have to scream at him, and at this point, he mimicked her screaming, and then he told her, "Just tell me, 'Simon, don't touch the flowers.'" Trying to contain Simon, Mrs. Smith found the day wearing and aggravating but a relief because while Simon's fits had always isolated them, now he was engaged with her.

This kind of interaction between Simon and his mother, in which Simon had tentatively moved out of the elaborate fantasies of his inner world and tested the actuality of his behavior against the real responses of his mother, seemed to have paved the way for more trusting and pleasurable interactions between them.

In other play with his mother, Simon picked up on the game of Shark Attack. Actually, Simon had ignored the game itself, but he was fascinated by the way the mechanical shark seems to eat the tiny plastic fish. At home, Simon assigned himself the role of the shark and when he chased and caught his mother, presumably eating her up, he was rewarded by being held and spun around. Thus, in play mother takes pleasure in her son's hungry attacks.

Simon was beginning to make physical contact with his mother, allowing himself to be occasionally comforted in her arms, and wrestling with her now and then when he tackled her during a game of football. He touched his mother deeply when he turned to her, some five months into the conjoint treatment, and said, "Mommy, I like being with you." At another point, Simon fell asleep in his mother's arms.

As summer arrived, Simon would ask me to fill a plastic container with water so he could extend his play with Eric, Ariel, and King Triton into an imaginary ocean. This container was just large enough for Simon to sit in, and in one quick and hilarious moment, Simon sat down in the pool, and just as instantly, he shed his clothes, and there he was, a nearly naked sea urchin, giving all three of us a great sense of pleasure and delight. This kind of play continued at home in the bathtub and outside in a plastic pool as he and his mother spent many enjoyable hours together. Simon's body was becoming the vehicle for relatedness.

In sessions, Simon often asked me to leave the room. I was permitted to stay when I acknowledged Simon's wish to be alone with his mother. A reconnection with his mother seemed to take place along other regressive lines. Throughout the spring and summer, Simon went through a period of intense biting, attacking his mother fiercely, often hurting her. Simon seemed to be posing another series of questions—similar to play earlier in the year—when he repeatedly asked his mother, "What will you do if I break this?" Simon seemed to be asking, "Can you take my aggression . . . can you take my hate, Mommy?" Once however, I interpreted Simon's biting along more joyful lines. I said something to the effect that, "Sometimes, Simon, when you bite your Mommy, I think you want to eat her all up!" Simon seemed to confirm the correctness of this comment when many minutes later he asked me what I did when he tried to bite me. It seemed that at such times I had often, as his mother had done in the Shark Attack game, redirected his biting by picking him up and swinging him in the air.

Simon created a variation on *The Little Mermaid* theme. At home, in a darkened room, with him and his mother in their designated roles as King Triton and Ariel, Simon, his trident temporarily replaced by a flashlight, arranges, again and again, for the sun to come up. This day, he tells his mother, "There is only good magic." He also requested to see a video of himself as a newborn and he asked for all of his baby toys. At other times, Simon would take his mother (sometimes his father) down to the basement, and while he would lie on her stomach, he would use his flashlight to indicate the birth of a new day.

Simon played these and other, obsessive, far less related games for hours each day, often the whole day, as he and his mother tried to recover their relationship. Simon often refused to leave the house, demanding his mother's continuous observation and participation in the intense but often obscure expressions of his losses, hate, and desire.

ATTACHMENT AND SEPARATION

At this point, some seven months into the conjoint treatment, Simon and his mother were making considerable progress in overcoming the impasse brought about by the disruption of their early attachment. The therapeutic environment had enabled Simon to regress and refind his mother, and, in turn, it had helped Mrs. Smith rediscover her son. Simon had established his mother as an object from whom he could seek both comfort and pleasure, and Mrs. Smith was gaining confidence in her capacity to provide for Simon. However, the picture was far more complex, their relationship, often precarious.

By making herself available to Simon's love, Mrs. Smith had simultaneously made herself vulnerable to his hate as well as his newly exposed fragility. Simon alternatively tortured his mother with furious and vicious attacks and frightened her with episodes of fragmentation and periods of despair. For periods, he withdrew into a world of impenetrable fantasy. Mrs. Smith's life with Simon at home and in therapy swung wildly among tender, although seemingly endless regressive play, incessant, shrieking demandingness, and bouts of implacable hate. For long periods, Mrs. Smith bravely contained this nearly impossible situation. At other moments, she felt her efforts were unappreciated; she felt betrayed and useless. She fell back upon the feeling that she was destined to fail—that she was a bad mother who could not do anything right. And Simon reinforced her feelings as he accused her repeatedly of being a "stupid idiot." Eventually, Simon's moods and sadistic attacks evoked her anger. On occasions, Mr. Smith could hold his wife and son; at other times, he withdrew or became enraged himself.

Another set of difficult issues were inaugurated by the process of separation. Having found one another, Simon and his mother were newly endangered by the threat of losing one another. Separations led to panic. Mrs. Smith's inexpressible yearnings for attachment and love had found their object in Simon. In turn, she struggled with her envy of Simon's connection with his father as well as with myself. Separation, brought about by Simon's anger or withdrawal, even, at times, by his growth, threatened Mrs. Smith with a loss of contact not only with Simon, but with herself. Simon surely reacted to his mother's conflicts as well as to his own. Feelings of connectedness seemed to frighten him with the actuality of dependence and the potential for loss and disappointment. In states of agitated fury, Simon coped by generating new visions of omnipotence acted out in identification with an assortment of magical characters.

The conjoint treatment continued for another six to nine months. Toward the end of this period the session time was often divided between conjoint and individual sessions as Simon was being prepared for individual therapy. We have discussed the first six months of conjoint treatment in some detail because we wanted to present a picture of an intervention that facilitated a regressive process. This intervention not only brought about the desired result of bringing Simon and his mother back into relationship with each other, but its achievement, in turn, created the basis for Simon's individual treatment and the slow, awkward, and fiercely resisted analysis of his dependence on his mind.

We leave off now the description of the conjoint phase of therapy, and keeping in mind the fact that Simon's relationship with his mother and father was followed closely, we return to the narrative of treatment with the focus on Simon. By describing three central games, we can examine in more detail the nature of Simon's defense, while providing, in broad outline and in a condensed fashion, a picture of the first three years of Simon's treatment.

As a precocious child, Simon had contrived an illusion that he was in control, that he could take care of himself. His most important relationship was with himself—with his mind. While his experience of the changes in his relationship with his mother opened up developmental possibilities, his experience of his mother's love was repeatedly broken up, destroyed, by envy and sadism and the ensuing withdrawal into the prison of his rigid, omnipotent defense. And, of course, he continued to be acutely sensitive to inevitable environmental failure. From this point of view, the therapeutic task was to find a way of communicating with Simon while remaining alive in the face of his destructive power and his need for absolute control.

THE TRAIN GAME

Four months into the treatment, recognizing Simon's interest in trains, I purchased, much to Simon's delight, a new set of brio trains. "I can't believe Ed got these new red trains!" he celebrated.

On one early run, his mother astutely asked him what the trains were carrying. "Milk," Simon replied. Simon's experience of nurturance, however, offered up in trains, toys, cookies, and attention was crosscut with profound feelings of loss, envy, and hatred, and fairly soon the enjoyable train ride was derailed. Simon would erupt in rage when his train fell off the track and he would destroy the layout. Occasionally, he would help me rebuild the tracks, more often he would insist that I do it alone. And so it would often go, I would connect the tracks, Simon would play with the trains for a short while, then he would destroy them, and then I would reconnect them. In between, he would wander anxiously about the room, finding nothing of interest in a room full of interesting objects.

During one such interlude and in a moment of architectural inspiration, I quickly redesigned the layout, adding many more complex elements. My effort seemed to intrigue Simon with a fresh sense of excitement, and we played for a relatively long time before the inevitable storm and subsequent act of destruction. But this time, when Simon asked me to reconnect the tracks, there was a new expectancy, as if my efforts were now somehow newly appreciated. A recognizable cycle of connection, disconnection, and reconnection had been created.

This emergent experience—this new feeling of relatedness between Simon and me around the trains—led to a series of interesting games. Simon's milk train became a passenger train and I was assigned the role of the boys waiting for the train to Manhattan, to New Jersey, sometimes to a barren desert, other times to school (Simon was now in nursery school). There was the bossy boy who demanded a ride—he often had to wait, the sad boy; he always got a ride!, the happy boy—who could endure the indignity of being last, the intelligent boy who could discuss the problems of the other boys, and so on. Sometimes we were referred to as the "lost boys." Simon frequently asked me to play the bossy boy and as I acted out this imperious boy's sense of entitlement and absolute control, Simon, recognizing his need for better self-regulation with his peers, would patiently but adamantly refuse my demands. As the play progressed I would imagine various conversations among the boys. The sad boy might confess the origins of his loneliness; the intelligent boy might reveal the burden of always being so smart. Simon listened closely to these conversations, and in this way, working within this metaphor, I could convey my understanding of him.

When putting together the actual train, Simon would insist on using all of the cars, so he would end up making a very long train that could not quite negotiate the complex layout that we had set up. What we believe we see in this aspect of Simon's play, that is, in his driven effort to take on mission impossible, is his attempt to demonstrate to himself his omnipotent sense of control. This was one source of Simon's continuous rage—he had to fail. It is, as if, in this scene, Simon had replicated his essential dilemma —a little boy facing and trying to master far too complicated a situation.

In one way or another, nearly every train game was inevitably brought to a destructive end. At first, in the early phases of play, a tantrum would erupt, seemingly without warning, and Simon would destroy the tracks. But, as the play became more organized, Simon would choose an action figure, and then this figure would destroy the trains in a violent wind and lightning storm. The boys would seek shelter in a fort and Simon as Nighthawk or Storm would attack and destroy the fort. As a representative for the boys, I would try to engage Nighthawk. Nighthawk finally explained himself: "He was mean because his parents had been mean." "How had they been mean to you, Nighthawk?" I asked. "They stuck a sword in my ear . . . another in my eye," Nighthawk anxiously replied. Such was the overwhelming assault on Simon's senses—the deadly impingements that had cut across his "going-on-being."

THE TRANSFORMATION GAME

There were many aspects of *The Little Mermaid* tale that had intrigued Simon and that were played out in the treatment, but it was the moment when Ariel, the little mermaid, changes into a human that we focus upon now. This transformational moment fascinated Simon. When his mother found an Ariel doll, whose fins could be taken off and replaced, Simon became a magician who continuously changed Ariel from a mermaid to a person and back to a mermaid. He was only slightly less interested in the moment when the witch-like Ursula changes herself from the huge octopus into a beguiling image of Ariel, as she tries to lure Eric into a trap. Simon became interested in magic and with a wand of his father's making he began magically to transform objects. For example, he would change me into a train, into an animal; once he changed me into the house where my office is located. "Ed is the whole house!" he declared. As Simon's interests moved from *The Little Mermaid* to *Cinderella*, he became enthralled in the power of the fairy godmother to transform objects. At the blackboard, Simon would ask his mother to draw a pumpkin or Cinderella's torn dress and he would wave his magic chalk wand and transform the pumpkin into a carriage and Cinderella into a princess. He played this game in the sessions and at home, again and again. In time, Simon became completely absorbed in an identification with the fairy godmother and her magical powers, and as an expression of this identification and the solution he seemed to be attempting, Simon began to dress as a girl.

Signs of Simon's interests in girl play were apparent before the first long break in therapy at eight months, but it was during this (vacation) interruption that Simon's commitment to doll play and cross-dressing deepened considerably. Once girl play emerged, it dominated treatment and family life for slightly less than a year. At times, during this anxious and stressful period, Simon seemed to be totally submerged in his identification with girl figures. Keenly interested in his mother's clothes, he insisted on dressing up. He once remarked that "my dress is my body." In a session, he imagined painting a dress directly onto his bare skin, pointing out that this dress would provide absolute "protection." Later, as he was working through this problem, Simon, emerging from a spell, as it were, volunteered that, at home, there was "one lady, one man, and one boy in disguise."

In sessions, while girl play was central, it was countered in nearly every session by boy play, that is, by the train game. Typically, in a session from this period, Simon would begin by painting or markering. This activity, which seemed comforting in its repetitiousness, seemed to be used to express and project destructive feelings. With his paintbrush or marker angrily slashing the page with red, black, and orange paint, Simon carried on (at times, aloud, more often silently) a dialogue with the various figures, Ariel, Ursula, and so on, who had come to represent the objects of his inner world. Eventually, perhaps no longer satisfied with the efficacy of this play to control the intensity of his feelings, and, no doubt to assuage the new anxieties that had emerged around separation, Simon turned to the Cinderella story, acting out in detail the drama at the blackboard or with puppets. My interpretations were refused, and increasingly, I was excluded, often violently. Literally, I was often banished from the room. However, when Simon finished this play, he usually turned to me and we would conclude the session with the train game.

At home, Simon's play with his mother was dominated by the stories of heroines. He could also entertain himself alone for relatively longer periods of time than had been possible up until this point. He would put on the tape of *The Wizard of Oz*, and, as Dorothy, twirl and twist to the songs that he came to know by heart.

At times, the transformation game seemed to be in danger of losing its status as a "game." That is, the identification threatened to become absorbed into Simon's personality and establish itself as part of his character. There, it might solve Simon's difficulties with separation as he found himself magically endowed, comforted by the visual and tactile sense of feminine things. At another level, it served as a "second skin" (Bick 1987), shoring up Simon's fragile sense of self.

What we would like to emphasize is the role of precocity in the development of Simon's play. Bollas (1987), in a chapter entitled, "The Transformational Object," presents the idea that the "mother is less significant and identifiable as an object than as a process that is identified with cumulative internal and external transformations" (p. 14). He suggests that the infant's first subjective experience of the mother is as a transformer of the infant's self-experience or state. We would like to put forth the notion that as Simon got to know his mother, carrying forward his first year of life history, he was fearful of submitting to her as a transformational object. In girl play he attempted to solve this need for the mother, first by omnipotently establishing himself as the transformational object—the fairy godmother—and second, by experiencing himself as the object of her care—Cinderella. In his game, Simon played both roles! That is, unable to surrender himself to his mother as "a medium that alters the self," Simon turned into the "medium!" Simon became not only the ideal transformational object, the fairy godmother, but the object of transformation, Cinderella—the little girl who goes from rags to riches. Underlying Simon's symptom—the wish to be a girl—there appeared to be a fantasy of total self-sufficiency.

THE WITCH GAME

Nearly a year into therapy, amidst the intensity of girl play and well after the train game had been introduced as a regular part of sessions, Simon discovered several puppets that were immediately established as the central figures of a new game. This game featured a witch's relentless and brutal attack on a somewhat befuddled king and his family. Importantly, Simon would often ask his mother to leave the room when we played the witch game, as I was often asked to leave when he played the girl game with his mother. In the case of the witch game, Simon, no doubt, needed privacy to express and work out the full range of feelings surrounding his internal mother, now fearfully and hatefully represented as the witch. And when, a few months later, Simon and his mother were able to let go of each other enough for Simon to begin individual sessions, Simon escorted his mother to the door, announcing that it was time for "men's work." The witch game, played compulsively in nearly every session, became the centerpiece of Simon's therapy. Thus, for the next two years, when Simon was not simply marking time with a board game, each session typically began with the witch game, followed by the train game until the train game eventually lost its appeal.

This internal family, "the most important family of all," as Simon eventually and perceptively referred to this motley group of puppets, is made up, at first, of a king and his son and daughter. Belatedly, the king marries his queen and eventually the family is joined by younger children and babies, at one point twins, a boy and a girl, a grandmother, and pets. Their castle is haunted by a witch who lives in the cellar, that is, underneath my chair. Not insignificantly, it would seem, the family began its existence on my lap.

The king awakens each morning, and just as he is about to make the day's pronouncements the witch emerges, giving the king a thorough thrashing about his head. "My, my," I, as the king declare, "it seems I start each day with a witch headache." The witch abducts the family and takes them across the room to the fireplace, a "dark, cold, and scary" prison, from which they can never escape on their own. However, they can be rescued, and another puppet, the "witch fighter," no doubt myself, is called into action. His powers are limited, however, and Simon eventually invites several Barbie dolls—the fairy godmother and her princesses—into the game to assist the witch fighter. Empowered by their magic, the witch fighter returns the family to their castle where they are permitted to relax for a brief period before the witch, having discovered that her prisoners have escaped from her dungeon, sweeps down upon them again, and the game begins anew.

In time, variations in this set piece were introduced that revealed different aspects of Simon's issues or demonstrated points of growth. Certainly, Simon's attachment to the Barbie dolls and his use of them as magical figures in the witch game allowed him the opportunity of enacting his fantasy of being a girl and brought the transformational aspects of girl play into the witch game. The fairy god-

mother—Simon always played her—was the only force truly capable
of thwarting the awesome power of the witch. He liked dressing her
and her princesses and imagined, at times, that some dresses were
more powerful than others. And when I offered to play the role of
the witch, Simon inevitably refused me, once acknowledging that
he "liked being the lady."

Simon's use of the Barbie dolls in his play provided me with a
good opportunity to comment on his identification with girls and on
the self-sufficiency that this maneuver afforded him. Once again, I
conveyed my understanding of Simon's play within the metaphors
he provided, and so I arranged for regular discussions between the
king and the witch fighter. These analytic observers readily appreciated the importance of such a powerful figure as the fairy godmother
in a dangerous world ruled by a witch, and the comfort the family
took in her help, and they were empathic, but, in the end, only to a
point. Later, they complained, often bitterly, that they thought they
could manage to deal with the witch and help the family without the
use of her magic. They also pointed out what they considered to be
the witch's envy of the enjoyable side of the family's life, in general,
and her fear and envy of the boy's aggressiveness, in particular.

The split in Simon's inner world was evident in his presentation
of the two idealized and grandiose figures—the witch and the fairy
godmother. At some point, he began to bring together these oppos-
ing representations of the mind—the tyrannical and the adored—when
he turned the fairy godmother into the witch and vice versa. The
family was amazed and confused, of course, relieved to be helped
by the fairy godmother, but frightened that they were actually being
seduced by the witch. Ultimately, Simon allowed me to play the witch
in this game, and I, disguised as a princess, would entice each member of the family to join me, but Simon, identified now with the
family's need for protection, exposed my true character and banished me from the kingdom.

The children in the family became increasingly important. Recognizing my own exhaustion at playing this game again and again,
a victim myself of Simon and his witch's inexhaustible supply of
hatefulness, I began to speak up for the younger children, convey-

ing how overwhelming it was for them to live in a world that offered them so little protection. We tried to hide, but the witch, with sadistic glee, found us and blasted us off to jail. At some point, the plight of this little girl and boy affected Simon, and he demonstrated, once again, the solution that he himself had adopted: he abruptly and magically changed the younger children into older children! Apparently angry and disdainful of the neediness of the younger children, he threw them, now older, back into the fray with irritation and disgust.

In other games Simon sent the children off to school where they were able to come and go, relax and learn before the witch ineluctably attacked them. Simon addressed his precocity more directly when the children practiced the piano. The witch was forgotten as the children attempted to play their pianos for the king and queen. Their parents, apparent perfectionists, became angry if their children made mistakes. They were not able to appreciate the witch fighter's advice that perfectionism inhibits their children's freedom and spontaneity. Simon took great delight in this mutually discovered game, especially when the children purposely misplayed in order to upset their parents. When the parents overreacted they were "penalized" and sent away.

There was a relatively long period in which the familiar routine was altered by a different sense of physical ease and pleasure in Simon. This feel of Simon's bodily accessibility was accompanied by a release from various symptoms such as lip licking or coughing, at least for a while. In his play, Simon sat in my chair—the back reclined—amidst the family of puppets, at one with them. I would sit next to him, on a footstool, with the distinct feeling that I was administering to a baby lying in his cot, his toys spread out about him. Here was a glimpse of the future boy, unencumbered by his mind.

THE MIND AS AN OBJECT

There were thus exciting periods when a new variation in the witch game was introduced and worked out, but this kind of excitement was often followed by periods of tedium as the new theme was sub-merged to the overriding requisite of control. A point to be under-scored is that the witch game was played by Simon with minimal variations for an extended period before he or I was able to intro-duce changes. Its potential as play was, in general, trapped by the maddeningly obsessive manner in which Simon rendered the basic drama. Thus, this game, not unlike Simon's other games and ac-tivities, was *itself* a by-product of Simon's use of his mind as an object. In the witch game, Simon did not simply present his internal world—he obsessively used the game itself to control primitive anxiety. Accordingly, in the transference, the game was used to manage his fear of me as a bad object as well as his contempt for me as a use-less object. Simon, as a true self (a psyche-soma), was imprisoned by his mind's frenzied commitment to an internal world ruled by omnipotent objects. He once said to me, in a manner that was at once cold and off-handed, "I rule this game." And, ironically but pertinently, I found myself affected by headaches and body tension as I tried to turn his mind games into a medium of relatedness. No doubt, I was feeling some of the despair and frustration that he felt "inside" his object relation.

In time, as Simon permitted me to offer variations in the format of the witch game—to introduce, for example, the piano game or to speak up on behalf of the children's "innocence" (see Shabad and Selinger, Chapter 10), in effect permitting me to use my knowledge to understand and help him—he was allowing another mind to in-teract with his mind, an occasionally joyful, and often, a very funny, commingling. This little boy appreciates a joke.

Simon accepted these interventions as my contributions did not challenge his integrity; I was ever aware and gave voice to his self-states. While, for a long time, I remained very much a delegated part in his mind, with no independent license to exist, his growing trust and affection allowed him to give me increased freedom to speak and be heard.

By accepting his control of the games, and yet moving within the metaphors he provided, I presented Simon with another point of view—another mode of experiencing. We thus began to construct a paradigm of interrelatedness within the confines of an object relation that had heretofore been designed to eliminate mutuality. What was in the beginning only a mind object for one—carefully cultivating its omnipotent narrative creation—has become an object for two as the story has gradually developed into a shared object. My acceptance and tolerance, at first, of a puppet-like experience mirrored this boy's own experience of his early life, which he believed was directed at him by external factors. I would have remained—as was Simon—only a kind of inmate to such a schizoid solution, but the pleasures of interrelating eroded the sole attachment to his mind as an object.

REFERENCES

Bick, E. (1987). The experience of the skin in early object-relations. In *Collected Papers of Martha Harris and Esther Bick*, ed. M. H. Williams. Perthshire, Scotland: Clunie.

Bollas, C. (1987). *Shadow of the Object.* New York: Columbia University Press.

Fraiberg, S., ed. (1980). *Clinical Studies in Infant Mental Health: The First Year of Life.* New York: Basic Books.

James, M. (1960). Premature ego development: some observations on disturbances in the first three months of life. In *The British School of Psychoanalysis: The Independent Tradition*, ed. G. Kohon. New Haven: Yale University Press.

Winnicott, D. W. (1965). New light on children's thinking. In *Psycho-Analytic Explorations.* Cambridge, MA: Harvard University Press, 1989.

5

Mental Interference

Christopher Bollas

Helmut lies in bed. It is 8:30 in the morning and although he has slept at times throughout the night, his mind has been racing. It is hard to recall what exactly he had been thinking about. He could recall pondering a conversation with his brother, who had told him with earnest affection that he should start up business as an ice cream vendor. He had replayed this conversation many times. He had imagined applying for a license, looking for a van, reading up on the production, which should be so simple, but well . . . he just did not know. He could see his brother's love and exasperation. His brother's face haunted him. But where would he go to find a van? Where do they make them? What would his friends think of him sitting in the van? Perhaps he should hire somebody to do that side of the business. He could try to set it all up and then hire a person. But if he did that, then how would he learn that end of the business? No one would be successful in a new venture, he knew, if they tried to run it from the top. One needed bottom-up experience. He found himself thinking of the colors of the van. White with a blue line around it? Blue with a white line? Did that fit in with the customer's association with ice cream? Maybe it should be red with white lettering. What would it say? What would he call the ice cream company? "Helmut's Ices"? "The Flavor Van"? "The Ice Cream Van"?

What would people think? He imagined countless types of people all responding differently to the name. Increasingly exhausted by these considerations, he thought to himself that maybe the ice cream business was not for him. What did he know about it? Nothing.

Nothing at all. And he had read that it was controlled by the Mafia, which used it to launder money. What would they do to him if he tried to enter their turf. Scene after scene of his ice cream truck being attacked occurred to him. They came after him in his home. They tried to kill him. They attacked and threatened his family.

The night wore on.

Helmut thought of other possible forms of work that night. He wondered if he shouldn't go into the retail sports world, concentrating on winter recreation. He had friends who lived in the mountains of France, Switzerland, and Italy. Long ago he had liked to ski. He envisioned opening a shop in London and one in each of the above countries. He would go in on the venture with his friends. How much, he wondered, would it take to invest in the setting up of such a business. He reckoned it would be probably about £75,000, and he thought about how much each friend would or could put into it. He recalled separate experiences with his friends, going over their recent times together. There had been problems. Some disputes. Ill considerations. He had gone out with one friend's ex-girlfriend and he had said it would be all right, but of course the friend had indicated that it was not all right. Then the ex-girlfriend returned to her former boyfriend—the now considered potential partner—and he wandered off thinking about their recent contacts and all the ins and outs. He tossed and turned in bed with each painful thought. The business brought him back to center, and he went back to thinking about sports stores. But he thought to himself that one had to be a sporting type and this he definitely was not. And he did not really like people. Or he thought he didn't. How do you talk to strangers who drop into your store? Anyway, what did he know about sports equipment? Where could he go to find out? He supposed he could spend a few weeks in the Alps and travel from one store to another. That was a good idea. He could see what they stocked and what he thought was missing. But how would he know what was missing? And what would they come to think of him if later he set up shop in competition with them and recollected that he spent time hanging around their stores and not buying anything. Thus he would have to purchase something in each store. That means he would have to rent a large car, a four-wheel-drive van, but what would he then do with all the stuff he purchased?

As the clock ticked through the wee hours he became even more exhausted by his thoughts. He moved from one job to another. From the travel business to the local recreation business. From the life of the dropout, just painting or doing ceramics, to a middleman bringing people together who could do business. This night was no different from all other nights. He dreaded going off to sleep and stayed up until one or two. He knew that although he would drop off for ten or twenty minutes, he would wake up again and then he would be launched on this endless journey of rumination. Yes, he would, he thinks, usually fall asleep, sometime around six in the morning, and get a few hours of sleep, but then he would awake again, and another struggle would ensue as he would try to find some way to get back to sleep, one strategy tried after another—thinking of a woman, thinking of a vacation spot, thinking of a recent pleasant experience, squinting his eyes to force stars and trying to disappear into sleep through them—but nothing ever worked.

He would lie in bed between nine and noon just thinking. It was always the same and went like this:

Oh God, I'm awake for sure. I can't go off to sleep again.

Well, get up then.

Why?

You have to get to work.

I don't want to go to work.

That's not a good attitude.

But there is no point. We aren't doing any business.

That's because you don't try.

Okay. I don't try. Maybe I should get up . . .

Yes. Get moving. Come on. Up and at 'em!

I don't know.

Come on. You can do it!

I suppose I could.

There you go. That's the spirit.

But.

But what? There you go. Getting down in the mouth again.

But what is the point? I will just get to the office. The car business stinks. My brother will only be embarrassed.

Business isn't great, but someone out there is selling cars. Why shouldn't it be you?

I can't work. I just sit and stare out the window. I don't answer the phone. I stay away from people. I have a sick feeling in my stomach.

You are pathetic. Absolutely fucking pathetic. You are just lying here in bed, feeling sorry for yourself, doing fuck-all, when you should get out there and work.

I am pathetic. It's true. What's the point in living?

Oh! Oh! So it's suicide time, is it?

Why not?

So if you can't get out of bed, and you feel like not working, it's time to just kill yourself?

I would be doing everyone a favor.

Oh, sure. Your dad, your brothers, your friends. They would be all delighted.

No. But they would get over it.

That's considerate.

I should do it.

Well, fuck you anyway. You haven't even got the balls to kill yourself. So how would you do it?

Well, I could jump off a bridge. But I suppose if I did that . . . well, I might still be alive when I hit the water and funnily enough I don't like the idea of floating in cold water, half alive. Um . . .

You're not going to kill yourself.

Or I could take pills. I could take a lot of them and do it. . . . Well, not in my flat, because I would not want my brother to be shocked. I could go to a hotel, although then the cleaning lady would find out. . . . I could try it in my car.

[This script goes on and on.]

Okay, so I'm not going to kill myself. Oh God, I suppose I should go to work.

Well, you've pissed away half the morning. Damn right you should go to work. Get up and shower.

I should do that.

Get moving then.

I'll count to ten and then do it. 1, 2, 3, 4, 5, 6, 7, 8, 9, 10.

Well?

I just can't do it.

Can't do what?

I just can't force myself to get out of bed. Maybe my brother will telephone me and then I will have to get out of bed. That's it, I'll wait for him to call.

What a pathetic creature you are. And you want to start a business. You can't even get the fuck out of bed. You aren't even worth a shitload of thought. Go on, lie in your own lazy excrement.

But what am I supposed to do?

Get up!

I'm too depressed!

You are depressed because you don't do anything!

No. I don't do anything because I am depressed.

This is only a small sample of Helmut's inner conversation as he lies in bed for hours. Eventually he gets up, although it is never clear to him what sponsors the gesture. He is exceedingly exhausted and first thing when up he stares at himself in the mirror, and for a few minutes engages in another conversation about how badly he looks. Worse than yesterday? Better? Signs of deterioration? So bad he should stay home? Off-putting? And so it goes. In the course of showering, without exception, he cries. He calls out, "Father, please save me," and in so doing he comes apart. But after this cleansing, he towels off, makes some coffee, and then has a bite to eat.

There is another battle that can transpire over fifteen minutes or another two hours about what he should do. Should he call his father and brother—who own and operate the used car lot where he works—and tell them that he is ill and cannot come to work, or should he bite the bullet and go to work? A long conversation can then ensue about his worth on the job. If he shows up to work—often after midday—he will retreat to his office, and spend the entire day wondering about his worth and whether he will ever sell a car.

He is 35. Tall, blonde, lazy green eyes, rather handsome. Catholic, but not practicing. He has been hospitalized three times since mid-adolescence. At 16 he began singing in a shopping mall and was arrested. It was unclear whether he was just high on drugs—which he took throughout his teens and into his twenties—or whether he was also independently crazy. He was released from the hospital after three months. In his early twenties he had another breakdown, this time unaccompanied by euphoric dissonances, but clearly a depression of some kind. His last hospitalization, some two years before he came to see me, was more preventive. His G.P., his father, his three brothers, and his family's priest all thought that he was "on the verge" again and more out of a wish to protect him, they put him into a private hospital for a week. He seemed, they thought, a bit better, after his release.

The family had met again a few weeks before I saw him. His father had a sort of sixth sense about him. He was pretty sure he could tell when Helmut was losing it, and he met with the G.P. in Helmut's presence. They had a calm, even congenial, conversation about how to handle Helmut this time, and hospitalization seemed perhaps a good idea. But the G.P., who was quite experienced and thoughtful, was less than content with this notion, and after considerable bargaining with the father it was agreed to give Helmut "a shot" at psychotherapy. The G.P. had never put the patient on medication, not because he was averse to doing so, but for some reason he thought that Helmut was the sort of man who once on medication would stay drugged for life, and he wasn't sure this would affect him in any event. There had been only modest outcomes from the medication he received in the hospital. The G.P. made the referral and said that he was quite sure that Helmut was unanalyzable, and he was not sending him along for analysis. But he hoped that Helmut might gain some minimal insight into himself so that rehospitalization could be avoided, and perhaps he could even begin to find his way in life, with some sort of jump start or nudge.

When Helmut came into the consulting room for the first session I found a man who was more of a vulnerable "kid" than an adult. He repeatedly smiled throughout the session in a kind of forced way, trying to put on a good expression. But he was also clearly anxious and almost stuporously depressed, and as I told him so, he seemed even more confused by my, as he admitted, accurate identification of his feelings. I asked him how he felt about attending the session and he said that as all else had failed he was willing to "try anything," but when I went silent he asked me if I could please ask him questions—he found it easier. He asked me how one spells psychoanalysis and what it was. I explained how I worked and lapsed into silence, whereupon Helmut said that he might just as well then tell me about himself.

He described his problems sleeping and the way he thought throughout the day, which I have tried to partly capture in the descriptions above. He occasionally showed up at the used car lot, but usually stayed at home. He described the several ventures he had tried in the last few years—selling small sailing craft, self-defense alarms for women, and a credit card security system—but each attempt had been less than halfhearted and all that he accomplished was the loss of £60,000, so that now he had virtually nothing left.

I saw him in twice-weekly psychotherapy for a year and half. The sessions were strikingly similar. He would report at length on his paralysis at work or in the home. As he described his inability to work he spoke of himself in critical and denigratory terms. I said that I could see why he found it so hard to work, as with such a critical voice within it would be hard to accomplish anything. He admonished me and told me that it had nothing to do with his inner voice, which if anything was helpful; but it did have to do with a defect in his personality, as he was unable to respond to perfectly reasonable urges from within himself. He said that he was disappointed in psychotherapy because he expected me to tell him what to do and to side with the part of him that did the same. But I didn't do this and this worried him. Instead I was silent too much of the time, and this was a waste of his time, and what he needed was tough questioning and my expertise. "I don't know why Dr. X. sent me to see you, but you are meant to be an expert, so I have come along, but I don't understand any of this."

He was puzzled by my affirmation of his feelings. I said that at least he seemed convinced of one thing, and that was that he felt uncomfortable in my presence and did not think psychotherapy would help him. I pointed out that this seemed to be the one thing he had managed to have unequivocal feelings about. He caught the humor in this all and said that he could see, then, how psychotherapy was helpful, as it allowed him to have a firm belief in something. He then proceeded for some weeks to talk to me *outside* of the psychotherapy structure, in that he would try to talk to me about his life assuming now that psychotherapy had failed, but that we should now talk about what he could do next. He continued to see me because he had promised the G.P. that he would stick it out for six months and so he would, as I said, fulfill his "sentence."

In the first sessions of his psychotherapy he told me that his mother had died when he was a baby—he didn't know how old, but he thought it was before he was 2—but he was sure it had not mattered and of course he could not recall her, nor for that matter any of the details of his childhood. Memory seemed to begin with adolescence.

As the months passed, however, and the six-month trial period concluded, Helmut decided to stay on for a while longer. There were several reasons for this. Listening to his long and deadening accounts of his internal mental life, I had repeatedly told him that with a mind like that–always ordering him about–I could see why he felt defeated. One session, when he told me that were it not for his constant mental approbations he would just do nothing, I said, "Really? You mean, if you did not tell yourself that you should do something, you really would do nothing? You would just sit there?" Yes, he was sure he would, for quite a long time, for a very long time. How long? I wondered. Two hours, ten hours, a day, two days, a week, a month? He was puzzled by the question. I said that he seemed to be living with a powerful idea that unless he constantly prodded himself that he would just be an inert heap, but personally I thought this was an impossibility. I bet him that if he let himself alone he would surprise himself by doing something. What? he wanted to know. How would I know? I said. It hasn't been thought yet, has it? It would just happen. However, to this bet I required two conditions. I said that so far as I was concerned, that if I were to be given a fair chance in all of this, I would need two very simple things from him. (As he was *full* of hundreds of demands, two simple requests struck him as almost amazingly reasonable.) I said that he had to come to psychotherapy regularly, whether he liked it or not, and further, that he had to show up at work, whether he wanted to or not. That was all.

What time should he show up at work? he wondered. I said it didn't matter to me. Anytime. But he had to show up every day of the week. (He had been staying at home and not working, perhaps putting in one appearance a week, sometimes missing two to three weeks.) He wanted to know what was the point of going to work if he didn't do anything. I said that this of course was the bet. I reckoned that he would do something, whether he liked it or not, but to do it he would have to be at work. The same was true of psychotherapy. He had begun to skip sessions, missing one entire week, and I told him that he had to come. What was the point, he queried, if it wasn't working? I said it couldn't work if he wasn't there. In any event, he agreed to this bargain.

Weeks passed. Quite to his surprise he discovered that indeed I was to win the bet. He found that if he simply arrived at work and sat at his desk, although an entire day could and sometimes did go by without his doing anything—not answering the phone, not opening letters, looking out the window—that two such days did not occur in succession and he would *just do something*. He would walk out onto the car lot and suddenly go up to a customer and talk about cars. Or he would go to an auction and watch the bidding. He would not bid as it was too anxiety provoking, but he learned a bit each time he would see how people valued things.

As the weeks passed into months he found a particular set of consistent interpretations on my part useful. Each time he would launch into one of his self-instructional diatribes, I would say to him that with that kind of intimidation—I would often call it the sergeant major self—it was no wonder he collapsed in a heap of desultory inertness. To his immediate but eventually diminishing ripostes, "But what will I do?" I would reply, "Nothing." Nothing, that is, in response to such internal "molestings," which, I argued, paralyzed him and paradoxically—because they were meant to inspire him to action—sent him to certain inactivity. So just see what you do, I suggested. And that pretty much is what he did for several months. And now and then he would report in a session that he had done something and on occasion it would result in something, such as the sale of a car, or the finding of a new source of automobiles.

We can see, in this respect, how Helmut's mind, full of militant instructions, was at odds with his self. If we apply the concepts of transference and countertransference to the intrapsychic sphere, we could say that the mind acted upon him like some unempathic, thoughtless, and demanding other, which left the rest of him feeling inert, vulnerable, close to tears, and completely misunderstood. His response to the mind's split-off activities was to collapse in its presence. Indeed, we were beginning to see that in fact he fought back by refusing to do what his mind ordered him to do, although such passive resistance was quite unconscious and only over time did he realize that a part of him was saying a quiet "fuck you" to the sergeant major. Work in this area was assisted, I think, by my attending to his differences with me. After an interpretation or a comment, about which I could see he had doubts, I would say that

I thought he disagreed; more to the heart of the matter, I would often say, "Ah, so you think, more analytical rubbish, eh?" and he would concur, eventually taking over this more generative critical response. In fact, his disagreements were often accurate and surprisingly informative, and led to a more constructive dialectic between the critical factor and its object. We managed to enjoy these moments and the pleasure of difference was gradually, very gradually, internalized into his intrapsychic life, so that those battles that took place between the self and the mind became more like conflicts between two rather evenly matched selves, with the combats not unpleasurable, and no clear victor or vanquished.

After a period of psychotherapy I decided that Helmut could use analysis, even though I sustained doubts about how insightful he might become. The reason was fairly simple. Toward the end of the first year I could see another very important dimension to his depressive illness. His helpless states were sustained conditions of need, and in my view he was unconsciously calling for a maternal figure to come and rescue him and look after him. That figure had been the father, who indeed often did come to his rescue, by giving him money, by telling him he did not need to come to work if he did not want to, and by worrying about him. I told Helmut that in my view his collapsed self was like an infant or a small child who was in need of mothering rescue, which he had found in part from the father, and that therefore he was armed against his mind, because this mind demanded independence and motivation on his part, but what he desired was care and attentiveness. Such comments were respectfully received by Helmut, although I supported his vigorous belief that such remarks were such as to be expected by a psychoanalyst, but we were embarking on a new phase of work that in my view could not be accomplished in twice-weekly psychotherapy.

In addition I had for months been puzzling over the mother's death. It was clear that he regarded this as completely irrelevant and analytical nonsense. But no one in the family knew how she had died, nor indeed did anyone talk about it. Out of grudging respect for what he regarded as my intelligence, he had asked an aunt about his mother's death and she had replied that he should ask someone else in the family, which he took two ways: first, it confirmed his view that it was unimportant and not even significant enough to discuss, but second, he agreed that it was a bit odd, as if she did not want to tell him because there was something she did not want to say about it. Bearing in mind that Helmut was not an insightful person, and furthermore that he tended to simply recount his daytime events with little interest in what anything meant, I had assumed the function of occasionally "producing" an interesting idea, one that rather caught his slight interest, even if he regarded such ideas as really quite farfetched. In the beginning, simply to be curious about something and to believe that one had the right to look into matters was itself somewhat new to him.

He eventually agreed to begin analysis after a particularly difficult summer break. He had spent time with his family on the west coast of Ireland, and had fallen ill with some kind of flu. His father and his brothers had not only not attended him, but had pursued mountain-climbing ambitions and left him for two weeks, during which time he had a high fever and was hospitalized. In hospital he felt he had "seen the truth," which he took to be a "fact" that no one had ever cared for him and that he had always been deeply alone. This revelation occurred during a significant mood elevation. Out of the hospital, his deep insight galvanizing him, he rented an astonishingly expensive car, traveled all around Europe, hit the casinos in Monte Carlo, and spent £25,000. By mid-October he somatized the manic state into a form of Epstein-Barr illness that was to last four months. And he was "flattened" into a kind of depression, but still haunted by his discoveries of the summer.

My comments about his need for analysis had occurred before the summer break, but he was not initially agreeable. However, the events of the summer and his depression in the autumn now convinced him that perhaps he needed to be seen more intensely. It so happened that apparently coincidentally he began to ask questions about his mother and her death. The father had managed to divert him by saying that she had died of an asthma attack, but when I recommended psychoanalysis, and Helmut told his father, it was as if in the father's mind this meant that *now* the truth had to be told.

Visiting his father, ostensibly to discuss the arrangements for the analysis, Helmut's father greeted his son by saying he supported his embarkation on analysis, but there was something he wanted to talk to him about. He disappeared into his study and returned with an envelope. As he told Helmut to read the letter he broke down into tears and Helmut spent the next twenty minutes reading and reading again his mother's suicide note. His father told him that she had been a very vulnerable woman, that she had had several breakdowns, and that he had not known what to do about it. He knows looking back that he left her alone too much, that he should have sought treatment for her, and that the week of her suicide she had returned from the hospital, and he had just decided to look the other way, going off to work. She killed herself when Helmut was 19 months old. Helmut's oldest brother was 9, and neither he nor the other brother (5 at the time) ever discussed the mother's death, which whenever mentioned had been understood to be an acute attack of asthma.

I have left out of the account the fact that I had told Helmut that the family's reluctance to talk about the mother suggested to me that this might not have been a natural death. On one occasion I said to him that indeed—and of course I did not know—it could have been a suicide. When he discovered from his father that this was so, it added to a somewhat growing conviction in Helmut that my oddball ideas—for example, that there were factors in the unconscious that were significant—had some measure of truth to them. I said that given the uselessness of his own mentational advice to himself, I could well understand that he was not particularly keen on any mind's ideas, including of course my own. How had I come to my idea? he wondered. I said that it was a *feeling*, one derived from the fact that no one talked about it in the family, and also one I thought he conveyed by his absolute negation of her significance. I was careful to point out how feelings derived from certain facts of life, but equally I pointed out that a feeling without a validating context—such as the one he provided through his own investigations—was potentially misguided. From this moment he had a greater respect for my mind because it had been of use on several occasions, and he could see that although I relied upon feelings, I also needed more than a hunch to validate an idea. It felt safer to rely upon a mind that worked like that.

Beginning analysis was not easy. In psychotherapy, by looking at me, he felt that he could sense my interest or my lack of interest, and now he did not know what I thought or how I felt. Analysis felt like being cut adrift. In the first week he was close to panic and conveyed it. It was not that I considered him on the verge of a decompensation, but that he seemed to have no personal assistance to help him through the loss of the visual object. I said that his response to the visual loss of me brought to my mind the loss of his mother, and that at this moment he was, seemingly without *anyone*. He agreed that he felt that he was without anyone, but he said he did not see how any of this had to do with his mother. She was dead and that was that. This simply had to do with the fact that I was out of sight and he found it uncomfortable. By the second week his mind was racing. He had a hundred things to talk to me about, to fill up the hour. I said that it was interesting how he used his mind to help him fill the void created by my absence. He agreed. I responded, "Of course, I know you will find this typical of me, but again, my association is to your using your mind as companion when your mother disappears. I think we are seeing that right here and right now." This made a certain sense to him in that, although he still claimed that his mother's death simply was too long ago to have affected him now, he could see the sense in what I was saying. This was different. He had found a way to find sense in these interpretations, even if he disagreed, while before he had only found them to be off-the-wall actions of the analyst.

Our senses of humor helped us through this period of work. When I would make links like the above he would complain that I was being psychoanalytical again, and I would reply of course, and I would not want to disappoint him. Sometimes he would predict my interpretations and I would congratulate him and tell him that I agreed—he was right. Insight was now a kind of amusement, but not one that was gratuitous; it was something that he expected of me and that he looked forward to, even if he was certain to keep his side of the equation present by knocking down the comments each time.

For some time he had complained that his father—whom he loved very much—nonetheless usually showed a cursory interest in him. He did not doubt his father's love; it was feelable. But his father only seemed to ask after him to rather sort of take his temperature. "Are you okay?" he would ask, obviously wondering about his mental state. When Helmut replied in the affirmative the father would sign off abruptly. The father did not want to know more about him. This allowed me to make a particularly useful transference interpretation, as Helmut was characteristically abrupt when I would make a comment that was aimed at a deeper understanding of him. For example, once I asked if he had dreamt that night and in a clipped tone of voice he said, "Nope, nothing I know of." Moments later, while describing his father's way of cutting him off, he said, "You have no idea how frustrating that is," and I told him how he did it to me, with the father's voice. He was genuinely quite stunned by this interpretation. He had no difficulty in seeing the parallel, and although he was less than enthusiastic about extending it to a family principle of not wanting to know about inner feelings and thoughts, he accepted that this *was* in fact the case.

For several months he felt his plight more deeply. He did not think about his mother, nor his life history, but the discoveries had shaken him. He was increasingly aware that his brothers, like his father, had removed themselves from any insight whatsoever. Indeed, a pattern of paternal alarm occasioned by the slightest sign of depression in him, followed by immediate detachment upon reassurance, invited a speculation on my part: it seemed to me that his father unconsciously linked him with his suicidal mother. This helped us to understand the unusual concern in the father, the G.P., and other members of the family about Helmut's safety, as everyone had linked him to the death of his mother. It also enabled us to analyze his own dissociated idea that he might kill himself, a view that he had held since adolescence, one that he had conveyed on numerous occasions to his father, his G.P., and attending psychiatrists, but a view that had no conviction. He did not really want to

kill himself, he told me, nor indeed did he have any suicidal
thoughts, but with engaging naïveté he said, "But it could happen,
couldn't it?" It took time to work this through so that he could see
that he was living out his father's memory of his wife's suicide, one
that the father associated with her infant, and with which Helmut
had identified as he grew older.

Interpretations such as the above were not only helpful, but also
the first indications, for Helmut, that *thinking*—the work of the
mind—could be helpful. For years his own mind had been occupied
with militant injunctions and merciless adjudications, and he had
unconsciously turned against it, becoming a listless recipient of the
endless stream of berations, but defying it by embracing an increasingly vegetative existence. In turn, he became more dependent upon
myself and the analysis. In the first year he had frequently complained about the journey to sessions and when he began in four-
times-weekly analysis, on the couch, he found it unbearable and
unhelpful.

He had, for example, complained incessantly about the silence.
What good was it to lie in silence for four hours a week? he would
ask. What were we accomplishing? he wanted to know. Sometimes
I would say that I did not know what would come from the silence,
perhaps nothing at all. Nothing at all, he would yelp. How could
we justify silences that produced nothing at all? I told him this did
not worry me as I knew that in time something would eventually
occur to him spontaneously, and he would tell me. He protested
with more worry than anger, genuinely feeling that this was really
the beginning of some kind of end, and soon I noticed that each
session he played with blue tack—a kind of putty—which he pressed
and distorted between two fingers of his right hand. I said nothing
about this, but he mentioned that he always did it—it had only now
emerged, however, in the analysis—and had since he was a child. I
said it seemed to soothe him and he agreed, so he would lie in silence for quite some time playing with his blue tack, now and then
complaining that the silence was useless and that we were wasting
time. I have to say that I found his preoccupation absorbing and I
felt quite sorry for him. Now and then I would ask after his thoughts

and he would report ruminative goings on, but as time passed I remember hearing *for the first time* the bird song outside my window, and I noticed that I was now sitting in my chair in a restful posture, relaxed and reflective. I also noticed that he seemed much less fretful. And he began to talk about matters that occurred to him spontaneously: a dinner he was to attend that night and the thoughts he had about it, a woman he had met at a party the previous week, reflections on his father's way of treating him at work. As he spoke up, occasionally I would ask for elaborations or associations. Sometimes I would add associations of my own, and now and then I would make an interpretation. The point is that by the end of the second year of work Helmut was able to use silence, to speak up spontaneously when he had a thought that carried weight to it—rather than the impinging weightless obsessions of his split-off mind—and he listened to interpretation and used it.

We could say that through a subtle form of regression within the transference that he was giving up some of his inner self-states to the other who used mind to help sort out the feelings and to reflect usefully upon lived experience. To my way of thinking this was the analysand's symbolic[1] return to the mother who had not been there for him in the earliest months of life.

This period of the analysis gave us the working relationship that was necessary to understand the next stage of difficult work. As his dependence upon myself increased, there were occasions of sudden and virulent outbreaks of mental interference, in which he would panic and then assault himself with hundreds of recommended courses of action. As he did so he was even more helpless and in one session said that he was certain now that he would accomplish nothing and be a failure forever. I said that I thought there was an infant in him that in a way did not want to have to think or work and wanted looking after, something he was now experiencing with

---

1. The ego can symbolize a need by using an object as if it were another object, in this case using me in a sense as if I were the mother. Ego symbolizations such as this take place frequently in any person's life and express the symbolic through use of the object rather than substitution of the object. A thing does not stand in the place of another thing; the use of the thing changes the meaning of the thing.

me, and that this alarmed his mind, which as we know had to do the looking after for him as a child. (Early in our work I had emphasized the positive side of the mind's effort to pull him up out of infancy and childhood by the bootstraps.) But there was indeed a portion of him that did not want to have to do anything, and this inert vegetative self, I suggested, seemed to me the infant who was demanding that the mother return and look after him. He vigorously protested this interpretation in the beginning, but by now I knew that he had to deny all links to the mother. So by this time I would let him fully and completely express his protest and then gently say, "There is to be *no* memory of mother, no link to her, is there?" and this very particular comment unfailingly allowed him to reconsider whatever interpretation I had made. In effect a certain kind of resistance had to be worked through each time, before he could make use of analytical interpretation, but arguably such comments—the work of intellection—only felt safe to him if it took into account his aggressions, his needs, and his desires, and was adaptive to his self-state. Then he could use mind: mine and his.

The final part of our work that I shall report was his growing realization that his failures in life—he had been out of work for long periods of time—expressed his demand that he be mothered. As such these failures were understandable and psychologically sensible. They were no longer simply to be the object of attack. As understandable as it was, in retrospect, that his childish mind would chastise and berate him for being childish, he had used his mind as a kind of militant other that had goose-stepped him out of his infantile self. But with the coming of his adolescence he instantiated a rebellion against this mind object and refused its companionship, moving relentlessly back into an infantile state, but not one accompanied by a sentient other who understood where he was. That presence emerged with the analysis, and in turn, he was able to internalize through understanding a companionable part of his mind that took his infantile states into account, did not berate him, and indeed helped him. Characteristically, then, he would tell me in sessions of moments when he had felt helpless or simply rather inert and he would say, "Well, I just told myself that this was not going to last forever, and that eventually I would come out of it," or "I was on the verge of having a go at myself, but I just told that part of my mind to fuck off, and sure enough, after a while I did know what to do." Finally these reports of his inner contests faded away completely as the process was being accomplished within the unconscious and needed far less active use of the analysis than before.

As he realized that his helplessness was in fact a destructive protest I brought to his attention that years of day and night reversal—when he would stay up until the early hours—had been his way of protesting the absence of maternal structures in his life by in effect refusing any structure to his existence. It was only with this insight that he agreed to a more reasonable schedule of his life. Prior to this he had partied many times during the week, staying up on occasion all night, and had taken vacations on impulse. The result had been to weaken his ego even more and although I had always pointed to his lack of a structured routine as self-defeating, he had refused to take this on board. At this point in our work, however, he saw the sense in my comments and gradually developed a routine that ultimately he was to find very comforting and useful.

Helmut helps us to see how patients suffering from depressive illness experience the mind as a split-off other that is remorselessly attacking them. When the depressed person collapses into an infantile state, he projectively identifies into his "mind" all the adult parts of the personality, but because of the severity of the collapse, these otherwise potentially helpful parts of the self become so split off that they are virtually yelling at the infantile self to hurry up and join with the mind lest there be a catastrophic structural split. In ordinary depressions such a catastrophe does not occur. The individual may sink into helplessness and inertness for a while—a few hours or maybe one day or two at the most—and although the more mature parts of the personality may have been projectively identified into the mind, which berates the self, or into an other who is now the object of envy, eventually the person comes out of the slump, rejoins mind as a helpful processor of lived experience, and all is reasonably well. But the severely depressed person experiences a catastrophic loss of mind that increases in its hostility to the self as it incrementally receives projectively identified healthy parts of the personality. If as is very often the case—as with Helmut— the child part of the personality hates the mind because it is iden- tified with a growing up that is a growing away from an essential truth about one's being, then the person can sustain trench war- fare between the self and the mind.

Psychoanalytical language is inexact and highly metaphorical. Were we not to have a clinical context for the distinction between self and mind, then readers of the literature would be quite right to wonder what exactly is meant by a split between the self and the mind, as such terms in the very first place are by no means clear. But as always we are obliged to justify our language, from my point of view, by indicating how our patients can only be properly imag- ined and considered through such terms. And in the case of the depressive, it is striking how this person *makes the theoretical state- ment that the self is at war with the mind.* This is not the analyst's invention, but one of the most common statements made by the depressed patients, and as such deserves even more considered at- tention. I think it is a startlingly precise statement of affairs. The person, in his subjective sense of self, in his own core being, feels assaulted by his mind, which pushes him further and further into a corner. He sees the mind as something harmful and awful. He thus prefers to be asleep than to be awake in order to avoid the hammer blows of the mind. He may consider suicide in order to stop the mind from attacking the self. He will engage in long, ex- hausting, and futile conversations between his self and his mind, experiencing in this polarization the distinction between his private subjective state of being and the mind that opposes that being.

Of course, he knows that his mind is part of him. He can even, now and then, try to identify with it, and from the lofty superego heights of mental reproach he can even joyfully cast aspersions on the inert self, declared finally to be a thing of the past. But such moments are short-lived, although naturally they become the basis of the manic development that can last for months. Eventually, however, the person is back to square one with the mind attacking the self with renewed vigor and distaste. But because this mind is

part of the self, indeed known to possess some of the most important and essential parts of the self, it can become an object of envy
(Scott 1975) and the person can bizarrely enough come to hate what
is in fact his. This may give rise to that masochistic glee of the depressive who takes pleasure in turning the mind's attacks into a form
of pleasure, engaging in an intrapsychic war between helplessness
and intelligence, between cynicism and megalomania. Less obviously
but no less importantly, the depressive person is always mourning
the loss of contact with the generative companionship of the mind.
The mind in health is a useful and essential companion to the self.
Those particular forms of destructive views that emerge from the
idiom of the self, occasioned often by the precise lived situation, or
the moods of a moment, are processed by the mind—one that may
projectively identify such contents, but one that eventually is part
of the reconsidering process. The individual will feel, as a self, helped
by the thoughtful capacity of his or her mind—its storage of memories of better moments with the object, its capacity to objectify guilt
and consider means of reparation, its time sense that allows it to
soothe the self with the notion of a curative factor in life that will
assuage the self's more immediate interests.

It is interesting in light of these considerations to rethink the
confusional states of the depressive individual. As we know such a
person can seem quite lost. Forgetful. Inattentive. Easily distracted.
Loose in thinking. Perpetually muddled. If the mind is hated, then
such self-states become means of attacking the presence of the mind,
even if as we have seen they invite its attack. But more than that,
confusion is often an effort to defy the mind's intellectual acumen.
Confusion becomes a screen that aims to deflect the mind's attack,
and depressive individuals may embrace confusion in order to mini-
mize the precision of mental reproach. Of course, the self will be
the victim of a mental standing order, for example, "You are always in such a total muddle," but the self habituates to such crude
reproaches and hides its mental contents from more precise and
devastating attacks by maintaining the confusional state. Psychoanalysts have no doubt observed the difficulty in getting the confused, depressed patient to free associate. This is often due to the

patient's deep fear that he is now on the verge of giving the mind the material it is seeking as the object of its fierce attack. It is better, reckons the depressive, to be a silent wreck than to be an articulate conveyer of mental contents that will only render the self more vulnerable to attack. The analyst's impartial consideration of the free associations, including his analysis of the patient's moral interferences, allows free thinking to occur and in time helps the patient to see that his mind's reproaches often are very wide of the mark, as the free associations refer to feelings and ideas that are beyond the penetrating glares of consciousness. Unconsciousness then becomes a kind of newfound freedom in being and adds to the patient's sense that he may, after all, be in ordinary defiance of the moral reproach, as unconscious life is too complex for single judgments and moral injunctions. Here is creative muddle: out of the confusions of unconscious processes, new visions and creative reflections emerge (Milner 1969).

In the manic state the individual identifies with the mind as an omnipotent and grandiose synthesizer of all selves everywhere, and a separate essay could be written on this side of the equation: mind as object. For in the manic state the mind becomes the treasured and adored vehicle of a triumphant trajectory over the woes of mankind. But my emphasis has been on the depressive state and on depressive illness, in which the mind is experienced as an alien object that attacks the self, driving the person into a profoundly vicious state of victimization Psychoanalysis affords a unique and special treatment for the depressive individual as the analyst will have to encounter the patient's defiant hatred of mental processes in themselves, and the analyst's mind will be attacked and nullified. Eventually, however, the analyst can present mind as an interesting and sentient companion, one able to bear and indeed to invite the subject's fury and demand. When this happens the patient begins to present increased mental contents to the analyst's mind for their processing, gaining relief, and eventually coming to believe that the mind—that of the analyst and that of oneself—can become an essential companion to the self.

Helmut's victimization by his own mind in his adulthood none-theless reflects a tradition established, in my view, in his childhood when he developed his mind along precocious lines in order to compel himself out of absolute loss of the object. In Corrigan and Gordon's chapter (Chapter 1) we saw how individuals turn to pre-mature mental development as an alternative to the mother but where the mother is still present, and one can feel the brilliant and aggressive effect of their act of displacement. Helmut, however, did not develop a brilliant mind by any means. We could say, in fact, that he moved the mind along the lines of premature superego development, understanding by this term not the Kleinian but the Anna Freudian superego, as that part of the self that is meant to stand in for the parent in due time, as a result of identification.

Winnicott's distinction of the difference between mind and psyche nonetheless raises puzzles in people's mind. What does he mean? Corrigan and Gordon, in my view, have illustrated very clearly how the mind object displaces the other and how mental life in and of itself becomes the alternative to interrelating. I also think one of their patients, Simon, points to an important distinction between psyche and mind, one that I believe helps us to understand Helmut.

One of Simon's compulsive rituals is around the story of *The Little Mermaid*, where he assigns the role of the mermaid to the mother, while he alternates between being the angry King Triton and a greedy sea witch. The setting of the story is, in my view, an important signifier, in that it points to the world of the sea, and to the impor-tant period in human development of intrauterine life.

While Helmut was *inside* his mother she suffered two breakdowns and was hospitalized. The recent work of Piontelli confirms what I think many of us have always believed, that intrauterine life affects the neonate's early relation to the mother and indeed to his or her orientation to life itself.

But the uterine sack and the neonate's place within it also seem to me an appropriate biological metaphor of what Winnicott means by the psyche and the psychic, as opposed to the mind and the men-tal. Being held within the mother's body is the first and only complete integration of the psychic and the somatic, in which the inter-communicating between the mother's imaginative and emotional life, as we know, also affects her biological relation to the infant, who is in that moment the recipient of her psychosomatic coordination.

Winnicott's belief in the value of "essential aloneness," which is only meaningful when considered through the alive presence of the other, suggests to me that the origins of psyche are derived from the mother's psychosomatic holding while the infant is *in utero,* and this extremely important phase of our evolution constitutes a fundamental paradigm for the interrelation between unconscious ideation, emotions, gestures, and bodily being. If all goes well during this period, then psyche is established. There is already before birth a history of psyche in relation to soma, both as this is the nature of intrauterine life, and because this maternal integration is "taken in" by the infant in his own coordination of the somatic and the ideational.

Psyche, then, as opposed to mind, always suggests a paradoxical partnership with the other: alone and yet related. It refers to the part of us that is unconsciously coordinative of response to the other and also the sponsor of the spontaneous gesture. Psyche is the trace of the earliest form of relationship, one that blends the mental into the biological and the biological into the mental.

The autistic child has always seemed to me someone who is not just motherless, in the sense that he or she cannot be reached by the discrete helpful other, but also someone who has built a hard shell—as Tustin (1990) emphasizes—around the self, to represent the uterine sack. He seems to point to the petrification of being while inside the human other, turning the holding environment only into a container, and a metallic one at that.

By playing his game Simon tries to get back to the sea. He knows where he must go, but he can't get there by himself. However, he has a highly attuned clinician attending to all the elements and one can see here how intelligent therapeutic adaptation to a child's distress becomes not only a holding environment but also a transferential action, as the analyst gradually puts the child in another

place. Both are at sea. Immersed. Not discontent with the immersion. Corrigan's pleasure in being with his patient, his tolerance
for being at sea amidst a most profoundly mentally confusing set of
circumstances, reflects in my view an understanding of how psyche
must eventually emerge where mind has been operant.

To put the mind in its proper place there must be creative confusion in the individual's self-experiencing. Confusion—mingling—
of all the elements. A see change. Where matters are not seen so
clearly through the rigid markers of ritual games, but become
opaque through interrelating, silences, and affects.

It was when Helmut tolerated his confusions and the silences of
the analysis, when he gave up trying to get an understanding of his
immediate self-state, that he then gradually allowed for the emer-
gence of psyche, of that form of thinking that is the interlaced
mingling of the ideational, the affective, and the somatic. The psychic, then, as juxtaposed to the mental, is that part of us—ultimately
in my view what we refer to when speaking of the unconscious—
that is inmixed with all the dimensions of human experience and
that serves as the irreducible foundation of subjective experience
itself. The mind is a special agency available to the individual that
makes consciousness, self-objectification, communication, and the
search for meaning possible. Without the psyche, however, the mind
is nothing more than *cogito* in search of *ergo sum*.

REFERENCES

Milner, M. (1969). *The Hands of the Living God*. London: Hogarth.
Scott, C. Self-envy and envy of dreams and dreaming. *International Review of
Psycho-Analysis* 2(3):333–337.
Tustin, F. (1990). *The Protective Shell in Children and Adults*. London: Karnac.

6

Mystical Precocity and Psychic Short-Circuits

Michael Eigen

PRECOCITY AND PREMATURITY

Winnicott's False Self and Lacan's Imaginary Ego

Winnicott (1958, 1965, 1971) was concerned with precocious development of mind as a substitute for emotional maturation. He wrote psychoanalytic poetry portraying split-off mental organizations enabling the individual to survive, at the price of mounting deadness and unreality. He developed networks of terms (e.g., *caretaker self, reactive self, false self, splitting of the psychesoma*) expressing facets of alienation in service of survival.

Winnicott's emphasis is an instance of a more generic, anthropological, structural concern, and links up with Lacan and Bion. Lacan (1977) placed decisive importance on the premature birth of the infant. That the infant is born long before it can care for itself functions as a symbol of discordance that runs through experience. Lacan especially emphasizes the gap between what the baby sees/imagines and its inability to coordinate motor responses to keep up with vision. The eyes are far ahead of what the baby is able to do.

Prematurity is linked with a kind of visual precocity, an eye-mind nucleus of ego precocity. Lacan describes how the infant substitutes a visual image of self-completion for somatic streaming, awkwardness, and incompletion. An imaginary "I" takes itself to be more whole than anything is, and reads its own and others' desire in terms of megalomanic scenarios: ego worship in place of truthful struggle. For Lacan, the imaginary, narcissistic "I" is necessarily paranoid and aggressive. It is forever molding self and other in terms of ideal images that funnel larger subjective-intersubjective flows. The "I" is inherently violent, since it is dedicated to trapping self and other by its versions of experience (or versions of experience it identifies with).

Winnicott's reaction against gestalt psychology gains in richness when coupled with Lacan's picture of the "I" as overextending visual perception of wholes, units, outlines (a sort of *visual capture*) (Rodman 1987). Winnicott's false self can partly be described as a dissociated eye-mind pretending (or falsely believing) it and others are more whole, integrated, complete than reality allows. He writes of the positive value of unintegration, chaos, doing nothing, so that welling up of fresh experiencing is possible. When Lacan (1978) describes spontaneous outpourings of the unconscious subject as "pulsations of the slit" (p. 32), he connects on a verbal level with Winnicott's (1971) "ticking over of the unintegrated personality" (p. 55). Lacan's imaginary "I" or Winnicott's false self do not have the last or only word.

For Lacan the violent "I" conditions object relations, and is not simply the result of the latter. Bad object relations may exacerbate and give direction to "I's" violence, but no amount of good object relations can solve or end "I's" aggressivity. The "I" always will have a tendency to precociously close or alter or funnel experiencing according to its scripts. It will always read itself in terms of the other's desire and vice versa. It is in the nature of the "I" to do violence to life. It does not easily *let be*.

Winnicott's emphasis on parental provision of a milieu that facilitates true self evolution seems, at first glance, to speak against the inevitability of a precocious "I" that ruins things. But he also notes that no amount of good parenting can do away with sadism, although parenting may play a role in how constructively or destructively the latter is used. Indeed, for Winnicott, instinctual sadism plays a role in the true self's affirmative movement. The false self, like the imaginary "I," does not end, but is incorporated in the tensions of a growing personality.

Psychic Breakdown

Winnicott (1974) immeasurably deepens his own and Lacan's work when he portrays the repeated breakdowns the psyche endures in face of its inability to process its own experiencing. The infant subject or self undergoes psychotic agonies that the immature psyche cannot process. To a greater or lesser extent, one may give up on ever being able to deal well enough with equipment that produces states it cannot handle. One lives, as best one can, through defensive organizations that ward off dread of being overwhelmed by agonies one lacked ability to work with. It is as if the psyche is injured by its own states and by its own immaturity. As one matures, a second, or more adult or competent personality grows over the debris of the first, and one learns to hide evidence of immaturity, disability, and helplessness vis-à-vis disorganizing emotional tides. Thus we always develop too soon and too late: too late to endure our early agonies, too soon to process them.

I think Winnicott here stresses a deeper immaturity than Lacan. He feels himself into a more pervasive experience of failure than the gap between seeing and doing, important as the latter is. For Winnicott there is a primal disproportion between agony and incapacity to sustain and process agony or overwhelming states (recall that for Freud the primal trauma was flooding; equipment cannot sustain, handle, or keep up with states it is called on to undergo). Dread of environmental failure is the outer shell of a deeper dread of failure of one's own equipment. The environment tries to make up for what the individual cannot do (and vice versa), but never with more than partial success. We rely on each other all life long for help with agonies we cannot handle. The human race in its entirety is hard-pressed to handle the collective agonies it is ever heir to.

The state of affairs Winnicott depicts is less structured than
Lacan's. It is not simply a matter of tensions between different ways
of processing experience, but a breakdown of processing ability
(whether primary or secondary processing). To be sure, Lacan's
portrayals are filled with irreducible paradoxes, reversals, and allu-
sions to what eludes linguistic webs (the overturning of scenarios
by the banana peel impact of the real, or the mercurial play of
jouissance, the never-ending "ouch" and "yum" of things). Lacan's
and Winnicott's analyses do not exclude each other. On the contrary, they fill each other out. But it is important to note that the
abyss Winnicott points to is not the cut or bar in language, not a
gap between or within systems, or the wound of the real, or the
opacity of primary repression, but rather a *cataclysmic failure of
the psyche to live its inability to sustain dire agonies.* We are not concerned here only with misdirection or redirection of experiencing
(metonymy and metaphor), but loss of capacity to experience, because the capacity to process (sustain) such a capacity was lacking.

Malevolence, Deficit, and the Embryonic Self

Bion complements Winnicott and Lacan. His work can be viewed
in part as a meditation on the psyche's inability to tolerate experiencing (precocity is substituted for experiencing). Bion delineates
at least three modes of intolerance of experience, which I am here
summarizing with the terms *malevolence, deficit,* and *embryonic self.*

Malevolence

Malevolence has a long biography in Bion's *oeuvre*, stretching
from his early to late psychoanalytic writings. It would be too much
to give a full account of this evolution here, but some mention of
facets of his work will be helpful. He depicts ways that hate attacks
links between thoughts, between feelings, between thoughts and
feelings, between self and other, and between mind and body. Something in personality cannot stand linking processes.

In early essays Bion (1967) depicted the attacker as a precocious superego taking the place of ego development. A warped, malevolent, hypertrophied superego preempted and usurped ego functions. For example, a moralistic life-condemning tendency left no room for thinking. Hate filled the gap where thinking might have been. Bion meant more than paralysis of secondary-process thinking. Indeed, secondary-process thinking is often commandeered by a moralistic, life-hating superego to justify destruction. As his work evolved, Bion depicted ways that destructive tendencies aborted or warped processing of affects at their inception. Malevolence can damage the psychic apparatus, so that metabolization of traumatic impacts is not possible. That is, primary-process thinking can be damaged, as well as higher level cognition.

The breakdown and reworking of traumatic impacts into material suitable for dreaming can be stifled, or poisoned, or deformed. A crippled primary process cannot begin the transmutation of raw trauma globs into usable feeling/imagining/thinking flows. Raw, unprocessed and unprocessable trauma globs, together with shards of aborted, deformed thoughts-affects (scraps of failed psychic movement), agglutinate and further block possibility of movement. One may depict this state as stagnant, as a graveyard or garbage heap— a dead or inert or wasted psyche. Yet malevolence gives this graveyard an eerie gleam. The psyche is at once dead and radioactive; its deadness takes on a poisonous life of its own, contaminating and destroying whatever comes near.

It is not just thoughts, feelings, and sensations that are deformed. The space where sensing/feeling/thinking might have been is altered. Instead of openness, a black hole. Instead of intensity, annihilating explosiveness. Not only space, but time is degraded. The personality condenses into a demand for everything now, so that anything that takes time is impossible. The little the analyst has to offer is rejected, because it is not all at once.

Intolerance of time and space makes it impossible for life (or analysis) to build on itself. Bion developed a grid depicting evolution of psychic processes. As a metaphor for massive destructiveness, Bion imagined the grid working in reverse. Instead of feeding trauma into primary process, where traumatic impact may be worked into images, which give rise to symbols, which give rise to thought, a stunning reversal occurs: any achievement gets deconstructed back into originary trauma elements, which remain unprocessable. Raw, everlasting catastrophe takes the place where a psyche might have been. The psyche (what there is of it) becomes a "catastrophe machine," grinding any bits of possible experiencing into horrific nothingness.

The primary task in personality growth is permanently undone. Bion (1965) writes, "The earliest problems demanding solution are related to a link between two personalities" (p. 66). Far from being able to "solve" linking problems, the personality set in destructive mode cannot even sustain them. It gets rid of them, attacks them, implodes-explodes them. Finally, it ends problems by getting rid of itself. In one of his most dramatic portrayals of destruction, Bion writes of "a force that continues after . . . it destroys existence, time and space" (p. 101). Annihilation goes on in subzero dimensions, even after destruction of personality. Bion does not offer a causal account of how such a destructive movement gets started, but once under way nothing escapes it. Malevolent precocity does not give the psyche time or space to develop.

Deficit and the Embryonic Self

Malevolence often masks and is triggered by a sense of deficit. Malevolence may even damage the psychic apparatus, so that it creates or adds to defective functioning. Nevertheless, *inability* has a biography in its own right, and cannot be understood merely as a cause or effect of malevolence.

Psychoanalysis usually understands *deficit* to refer to some lack or ill in environmental provision, a deficiency in personal or social nutrients necessary for growth. Bion does not exclude this, but his concern is broader. He calls on us to face the fact that our ability to process experience is not up to the experience we must process. This is not only so in infancy, but all life long.

Difficulties inherent in tolerating and processing experience cannot be written off as malevolent attacks against aliveness or failure of environmental provision, although these are important. We come against limits, walls, holes in processing ability every step of the way. Part of failure of provision reflects a general difficulty human beings have in working well with their own and others' experience.

Bion attributes part of our deficient processing ability to the embryonic nature of self, psyche, mind. If our mental apparatus evolved in service of survival (adaptation), it may be ill-equipped to handle issues of integrity or emotional truth, important later in our history. Our capacity to work with tensions between integrity and adaptation may be embryonic. The tension between conflicting claims may give rise to new ways of being a person. The very idea of what it means to be a person may be embryonic, in process of development, getting ready to be born.

We must make room for the idea that we are eternally embryonic. Perhaps our ability to do *any* experience justice is embryonic, the more so our ability to make the most of conflicting experiences and approaches to experience. The idea that we are embryonic takes the edge off deficit. If we are embryonic, there is hope we may grow. The embryonic self carries the possibility of becoming, an ever-open *not yet*. Yet it is important to note that Bion does not have a utopian idea of growth. No amount of growing and learning will supplant or eradicate the permanent embryonic dimension of living.

Neither the malevolent self nor the embryonic self exhausts the area of deficit. A hallmark of defective hardware, equipment, or mental apparatus is an incapacity to let experiencing build. As noted above, this runs deeper than failure of secondary process. For Bion, the capacity to let experience build begins with the transformation of an impact into dream work, myth, symbolization, affective images, and primal narratives. The deficiency in our equipment begins whenever processing of experiencing begins, a primary-process deficiency. We cannot keep up with experiential impacts. Production of experience outstrips assimilation. Our equipment produces states it cannot handle. It is doubtful we can ever catch up with ourselves, or do ourselves justice, whatever level of processing we tap.

We are too much (or too little) for ourselves. Bion amplifies ways we cannot support ourselves and each other. We get rid of, evacuate, shunt, or turn off our experiential capacity, our sensitivity. This may involve destructive and embryonic processes, but in principle goes beyond them. The inability to support ourselves is built into the way we are together. If we do not make room for inability to support ourselves and relationships, if we do not make room for deficit, we place too great a burden on what we *can* do. We may try to do too much, overextend ourselves, substitute omnipotence for openness, ravage ourselves with mastery rather than discover what partnership can mean.

Summary

We have linked precocity of ego development with the infant's premature birth. Aspects of ego functioning outstrip the slower, more gradual development of psychomotor coordination. Image outstrips ability. We wish we could do things we can't. As infants, and all through life, we imagine ourselves able to do what we see others doing. There is a gap between what we see, imagine, wish, and true achievement. There is an *eye-mind* we can never keep up with.

The time lag between and within our selves also has deeper roots. The impact of trauma, and emotional experience in general, is often too much for our equipment to process. We are not up to the agonies that beset us. Our equipment produces states it is not able to handle.

It is easy to imagine an infant unable to process turbulence it undergoes. But I think it helpful to confess a processing incapacity all life long. Our religions and psychotherapies offer frames of reference for processing unbearable agonies, and perhaps, also, unbearable joys. At times, art or literature brings the agony–ecstasy of life together in a pinnacle of momentary triumph. Good poems are time pellets, offering places to live emotional transformations over lifetimes. There *are* moments of processing, pulsations that make life meaningful, as well as mysterious. But I think these aesthetic and religious products gain part of their power from all the moments of breakdown that went into them.

We have developed a rhetoric equating falseness with defensiveness, a rhetoric of the double, or counterpart, or substitute self occupying the place where a true self might have been. We picture the substitute self as a second self, more complete, less subject to breakdown, tougher skinned than the first. Underneath is pure sensitivity, without muscle, bone, or skin. At the same time we associate the originary, true self with wholeness, or with spontaneity and impulse. The substitute self is a kind of runner-up, what we make do with in real life in order to deal with hardship. Yet substitute pleasures make up for a lot, and sometimes are all we have.

We become diffuse by filtering our personalities through too many versions of self, and rigid if we take too few too literally. Part of processing includes symbolizing facets of self and relationships to self. We develop expressive forms for breakdown or ruptures in processing, and how we relate (or fail to relate) to incapacity. We symbolize, also, orgasmic-ecstatic moments, as well as the hard work of problem solving, turning things over, chewing on things.

Our communications impact on each other's sensitivity, setting off more processing work, some of which bears fruit. Whether we defend, modify, amplify, or deepen our positions, we need the work of the other to bring out our own. We feed on each other's work, allied processors, friends or enemies, at work together.

THE MYSTICAL CAPACITY AND SENSE OF RIGHTNESS

It is important to spend time thinking about the different states one goes through in a day. In one day, even a few hours, one may feel one with God, explode in fury, quiver in fright, weep, work hard at something. One may be a skillful hunter ready to take on the world, or roll up in a ball in bed.

Freud marveled at the plasticity of the psyche, its changes of state.
He felt this capacity held out hope for treatment of psychosis. If we
go back and forth from dreaming in sleep-life, to common sense in
wake-life, why prejudge what is possible, what transformations of
self await us? Meditating on our capacity to change states may enable us to be a bit freer from entrapment by any one state, and to
get as much as possible from the states we go through. Dwelling
with changing states deepens our inner-outer texture (our inside
rings grow, our outside bark multiplies ripples).

There is a mysticism of changing states. The very experience of
changing states can be highly charged, numinous. The amazing
diversity and extremes of experiencing can give rise to a sense of
awe and mystery. How can all we experience be possible? What sorts
of beings are we? What can we do with the restless palate that gives
life its colors? Surely we can do more than point and nod, as the
great display slides by.

Often the mystic of changing states is manic. His panoramic vision flies over vast psychospiritual landscapes, scanning for prey.
Now and then he swoops down and turns a few captured moments
into prayers or poems or plays or papers. Or he may gaze unblink-
ing into the vast shifting navel of vision and throw stones. Such a
mystic keeps shifting positions in order to maintain exuberance.
Every movement opens new vistas, new thrills. The passing years
leave no rings inside, no ripples outside. He is as blank at the end
as at the beginning, although his life may be in ruins.

The manic mystic short-circuits the states he spies. It is enough
to see them, to taste them a bit before spitting them out as aesthetic,
religious, or psychological products. The manic mystic is able to
avoid being changed by the states that thrill him. This is different
from the mellowing of the seasoned mystic, who is deeply affected
by what he goes through, and undergoes corrective transformations.

The seasoned mystic gets something out of the changes he goes
through, and does not merely luxuriate in hyperawareness of change.
He does not simply ride the waves, nor masochistically go under,
although he may do each at different times. He is brought up short,

revisualizes himself, rediscovers life where the real becomes symbolic, and the symbolic becomes real. There is a mystical agony when one sees everything wrong with oneself magnified to infinite power. One patient dreamt of this as a bug inside the pearl (Eigen 1992). The shock of bottomless malevolence, madness, and deficit brings one to one's knees. One hungers for truth about oneself, even if it is impossible to bear. The beatific vision is complemented by vision of one's ugliness. One needs input of both for balance. Both are real, both imaginary.

The vision of destructiveness (like destructiveness itself) can never be fully integrated, transformed, metabolized, processed, converted into something useful. Our ability to injure ourselves and others never ends. It is cruel to rationalize all destructiveness as secretly useful, as hidden good. I think we must make room for the possibility of destructiveness as such. Making room is not indulgence. Making room for the possibility of really being destructive, without precociously rationalizing it, makes room for spontaneous growth of protective measures. If one confesses one's viral (virulent) self, one's touch may soften.

This is not a matter of saying, "I'm sorry, I'll be good," or a matter of making resolutions. One knows such attempts spiral out. Being touched by vision of destructiveness (one's own, others', life's, the broader currents one is part of), cuts one to the core, makes one less hard-hearted. One becomes less harsh and strident and spongy. Facing one's destructiveness is no immunization, but it gives one a different smile and glance, a different "feel."

In a recent session, a patient (Dolores) with years of immersion in mystical experiencing, began speaking about losing the "analytic stance" in sessions. She was taking courses in psychoanalysis, and feeling bad about not keeping the analytic stance with her patients. Other therapists in her peer group were taking courses too, and sounding more analytic. Dolores was a very sensitive, gifted person. I found myself repeating the words *the analytic stance*.

Dolores was wounded to the quick. She furiously withdrew, cried, then attacked me. She felt I was making fun of her, putting her down

for not being analytic. As far as I could tell, I was trying out her phrase
for size. The analytic stance? I had visions of analytic pretentious-
ness I encountered over the years. Here was Dolores, so psychically
prescient, adept, intricate. Many analysts seemed crude and butcher-
ous by comparison. Was she measuring her ability by some pro-
crustean phrase?

After enough time passed to absorb some of the emotion in the
room, I remarked, "If anything, I was making fun of the phrase, not
you. What the hell *is* the analytic stance?"

It was a momentous event. In an instant, puff! Puff went her picture of me ridiculing her, her conviction that her rage at me was
totally justified. An instant visionary flash exploded all the times she
raged at the other, feeling justified by her sense of injury, never
doubting her perception. At such moments her vision of the other's
destructiveness threatened to doom her in an abyss of worthlessness,
which she raged against. Her sense of rightness was absolute.

"The analytic stance," I mumbled. "Puff," I trailed off with a wave
of my hand.

She laughed and laughed, free from certainty. We smiled at each
other, and felt the spread of feeling circulating back and forth, a
good permeability, free of sensitivity rape and paranoid rage. A prison
she hadn't known she was in momentarily disappeared. Self and other
could not feel quite the same again.

Mystical Moments

For Dolores, life was essentially mystical. So much of her experience
was highly charged. She lived from heightened moment to heightened moment. Life was cosmic drama with a cosmic glow. She moved
from union to union, suffering agonizing disruptions of union. As
often happens with individuals who possess a strong appetite for
union, she tended to live alone. Her aloneness heightened moments
of union, and gave all experience greater impact. Aloneness protected
sensitivity.

So much of her experience was organized around a nuclear sense
of rightness and certainty. She stayed close to what felt right for her,
and when she found what felt right, there was no room for doubt.
She was swept away by the intensity of perceptions, which were nearly

as absolute for her as a schizophrenic's hallucinations. For Dolores, perception was, as William Blake suggested, infinite. Thus, for Dolores, life was ever meaningful. Each moment was saturated with meaning. However, she did not recognize the attitudinal basis of her perceptions; she was not tuned in to the attitudes that organized the tone and slant of her perceptual world. In particular, she never doubted the rightness of her sense of rightness. For Dolores, what felt right was the truth of her being, her soul's verity. Above all, life was soul-feeling; what the soul felt *was* true, and what was true *must* be right.

For Dolores, life was orgasmic. Not just body orgasms, but feeling orgasms, soul orgasms, self orgasms, ego orgasms. Not all experiential impacts set off orgasmic fireworks. Dolores was an artist and actress, as well as therapist. She painted and acted soul feelings, so that states of being she lived and expressed were finely nuanced. Yet even when the volume was low, and gradation of feeling varied, life was an ebb and flow of orgasmic seas, with rising undercurrents.

Dolores *knew* life through the rise and fall of orgasmic feeling. Orgasm was a mode of cognition, a tuning fork, a magnet, a magnifier. It focused and heightened significant aspects of life. Through soul orgasms Dolores evaluated and tasted life more keenly. From the quality and feel of orgasm, Dolores could tell how good or right or wrong something was for her. Dolores read the taste and feel of orgasms (body-mind-soul-self-ego) for messages about her path. Orgasms provided destiny messages.

It had never dawned on Dolores to what extent she relied on the orgasmic sense to judge experience, or to what extent her ego was a judging ego. She had prided herself on being nonjudgmental, on living openly. Now, suddenly she saw a hidden connection between orgasmic judging and ego judging, how a judgment flash that had orgasmic authority closed her down. Just as she thought she was most open, an orgasmic judge pulverized whatever person or moment filled or tore her.

Orgasm was a way of processing *and* obliterating experience. For a moment it took her closer to herself and the other. But then it turned, and the gap between herself and the other seemed unbridgeable, or filled with hurt and rage. The orgasmic flash began with sweetness and joy, but ended in fury. Lover and enemy were one.

The moment Dolores and I laughed together was free from judgment. If anything, we were gleefully judging destructive judgment,

perhaps a little like kids getting away with something. But I think
for the moment we found the capacity to play, to enjoy feeling alive
together, to simply flow. The prison of judgment temporarily dis-
solved, or partly became an object of humor, rather than a totally
gripping horrific reality. Dolores felt what it was like not to be gripped
by a judgment that had the authority of ego and orgasm, a judgment
that thrived on terror and rage. She found herself in an intersubjective playground bigger than the sum of parts.

MYSTICAL PRECOCITY AND
MYSTICAL MATURATION:
FORGIVING THE UNFORGIVABLE

Mystical experience can be used to further or short-circuit personality growth. As often happens, as was true for Dolores, it does both
for the same person. To what extent does it do one and the other?
Can we tip the scales more in one direction or the other? To what
extent ought we meddle with capacities we don't understand? How
can we get to know our mystical capacity better, so that we and it
may grow together?

We are not in a position to say, "I don't believe in mysticism,"
and turn attention to important, real matters. Too much is at stake
to be dismissive. It took less than ten years for a mysticism of hate
to end Yiddish culture in Europe. The swastika and goose step were
parts of a mystical surge, a military mysticism that cemented huge
portions of a nation. Words like *pure* and *super* played on echoes of
holiness, placing the sense of boundless transcendence in the service of precise destructiveness.

Dolores's mysticism didn't hurt anyone but herself. Her precocious
mystical capacity helped and harmed her. The gratification she got
from her mystical capacity held her together. At the same time, it
decreased motivation to develop her intellectual and practical potential. She barely made a living.

Most of her life she did not mind a threadbare existence, since
her life was filled with self-feeling. Cosmic suffering and joy com-

mingled to make her life full, rich, meaningful. The moment was enough. As a young woman she enjoyed a mysticism of the senses. Sensation and sexuality held her together. She lived a kind of Tantric philosophy, a *Song of Solomon* existence. She lived like the lilies of the field, with no thought of the morrow, in God's hands. As time went on, mystical feeling spread through her body, and led to dancing, painting, acting. She was a body mystic, yet her eyes shined with earnest, loving transcendence.

As a child she felt loved by her father, although he was perceived as ineffectual in worldly terms. Her mother was near psychotic and Dolores had a psychotic sibling, and her other siblings had marked difficulties. One could say she lived her father's life in a transposed key. She became a version of father as refuge against mother. Yet Dolores was also very much an original, her own person.

Her mother wanted her to be an intellectual, social, and worldly success. Dolores was gifted and had the potential to shine. But she fell apart in college. Head learning tore her to shreds. She felt she could not and did not want to become the showpiece her mother wanted. She would *not* be successful, at least as defined in common, worldly terms. It was enough to just *be*.

Her mother was dismissive and invasive and incessantly plunged Dolores into dire agonies. Her father's love saved her, but could not make it safe to use the intellectual, social, and practical capacities that her mother desired. Dolores did what neither parent expected. She lived off a deep sense of mystical intensity that took her out of the family, into the river of life.

Dolores would be an eternal child, always young, always new. Yet she was rich with experience. Why did she seek help? What did she want from therapy? She had never wanted marriage, children, money, mainstream living.

She was a child of the cosmos, a daughter of the dance of life. What did she want from me?

Our first year of work was characterized by moments of intense connection, punctuated by the latter's rupture. Moments of high emotional-erotic-mental-spiritual arousal, which bordered on exquisite ecstasy, were repeatedly smashed. Dolores would become deeply wounded and incensed at what she regarded as my cruelty or insensitivity. This is a pattern that characterized her close relationships. One could relate it to various aspects of ruptured union with par-

ents. Her traumatic object relational history would be enough to
explain the repetition. The other alternately *was* loving, cruel, insensitive, implosive-explosive, vacant.

Dolores had years of therapy and my sense was that historical
"explanations" were necessary but not sufficient. As we went through
the *wounded union* moment repeatedly, I had the strong sense that
we were not simply reliving, but trying to create something new. Our
immersion in the wounded union moment allowed Dolores to experience the realness of both union and separateness, their swings,
comminglings, sorrows, ecstasies. No amount of therapy makes them
go away. They are permanent parts of experience. By our going
through them together, Dolores could gradually take them as part
of a larger intersubjective flow.

Our going through the wound together was different from what
she did on her own. With her parents the trauma was repeated, more
of the same. Our moments of trauma led to new possibilities of experiencing. We not only talked about traumatic impacts with mindful
awareness, nor simply enlarged our mental frames of reference, although these were important. Dolores's heightened reactivity to my
traumatic impacts on her had an enormous impact on me. Her sensitivity fine-tuned me. I experienced my wounding impact on her
repeatedly and thoroughly, and in subtle ways spontaneously re-
worked myself around her sore spot. I grew through Dolores's pain.

We are elastic and inflexible. No matter how I stretched and grew,
I had traumatic impact on Dolores. But Dolores saw and felt her
impact on me. She could change me, although not entirely. She saw
that I would have liked to have been different, if I could, and that
her influence, at least, made some difference. She was not simply
sloughed off, ignored. Through our interchanges I was becoming the
sort of person she could forgive, although I, also, remained unbear-
ably unforgivable.

Dolores's mother could not enter into interchanges that might
change her. She went on blithely beyond influence, vaguely omniscient and oblivious. An oblivious omniscient individual tends to be
helplessly enraging rather than forgiveable. Dolores's psychic flow
was clotted by *an unforgiving attitude stuck to an unforgivable object*. Perhaps some of her hypersensitivity was an attempt to burst
past this barrier. She could calm down somewhat with me because

her sensitivity affected my sensitivity in ways that changed my self and person. We discovered mutual sensitivity deeper than trauma. When I became someone she could (sometimes) forgive, my unforgivable aspect became (sometimes) more lovable or tolerable. She could put up with me because of what she got from me, what we got from each other. At least with one person, for some moments, the unforgiving attitude stuck to the unforgivable object could begin to thaw. Her perception of her impact on me enabled her to let down and experience her stiff and unyielding aspect, her "soul rightness" described earlier. My painful admission of my wrongness (how I could wrong the Other) allowed her to feel how wrong her rightness could be.

In so much of life, defensive rightness in one person triggers defensive rightness in another, spirals of defensive reactiveness. Dolores's mother could never be wrong about anything basic. She was never at fault, at risk. She could not live from wound to wound, sensitivity to sensitivity, unless filtered through defensive rightness. She was not aware of the rightness that stole responsiveness; she simply *was* right. Dolores had not been aware how much her sense of mystical rightness aped her mother's oblivious omniscience. She would have been horrified to think that her capacity for mystical experience shared her mother's blindness.

Dolores's capacity for mystical intensity made life worthwhile. She never focused on the rightness or judgmentalism of mystical vision. Mystical awareness was nourishing, enriching, fulfilling. It lit up existence. The blindness of mystical darkness was inherently ecstatic. That the mystical richness of life should have something in common with her mother's unconscious snobbery was unthinkable.

Without quite realizing it, I modeled the ability to feel deeply wrong in relationship to the Other. I gave Dolores a chance to experience someone feeling deeply wrong and sorry without masochistic surrender. This smoked out an incapacity to feel wrong buried in mystical rightness, an incapacity all too obvious in her mother's prosaic rightness. It never dawned on Dolores to develop a critical stance toward the sort of experiencing that enhanced her life, the area of life she felt certain her mother did not invade. If she was wrong about mystical experiencing, she was wrong about everything.

Mystical Awareness as Psychic Short-Circuit

Mystical states can short-circuit working-through processes. There are moments of beatific union with self or Other that bypass painful realities. One can wait or strive for such states instead of working with personal difficulties. Certain mystical moments are akin to being in the goal region without going through the maze. One enjoys the excitement and richness of the event, without worrying about preparation or cleanup.

One takes a direct, nonstop rocket to divinity, a mixture of sensation, feeling, intuition. Intellect is used mainly to drill deeper wells, or make better openings. One lives in and for these states, never far from ecstasy. One's cup runs over, filled to bursting with heavenly sensation and feeling. The divine moment leaves. One is alone, forlorn, in agony. One is terrified and enraged at the other's indifference, insensitivity, cruelty, incapacity. One feels grieved for life's wounding ways. Feeling disappears. There is deadness, emptiness. Then the rocket fires again. One weeps tears of recognition, gratitude. One's heart is radiant.

The cycle repeats with many variations. Life becomes a raw affect flow, a rise and fall of naked affects. Everything else is extraneous. The affects are, alternately, blessings and curses, cosmic portals. Through the rise and fall of self-God sensations-feelings, life is revved to infinite power.

I recall learning about rats starving as they kept pressing a bar that triggered electrode stimulation of a pleasure center in the brain. Mystical sensation-feeling can be addictive. Dolores's life was dangerously near the poverty level yet rich in cycles of feeling. The word *pleasure* scarcely does justice to the surge and diminishing of mystical intimations, mixtures of bliss, joy, ecstasy, suffering. One's life can be devoured by radiance.

Somewhere Isaac Bashevis Singer wrote, "God gave us so many emotions and such strong ones. Every human being, even if he is an idiot, is a millionaire in emotions." Singer seemed almost an ideological naturalist, yet his work teemed with demons and angels. He portrayed individuals who could not take the emotions or emotionlessness of existence. People's lives were broken by the mystical capacity that gave them meaning. Lives also were broken by lack of this capacity, by bleakness. Whether ineffable joy or terror, human equipment was not up to what it must endure. Neither mysticism, nor lack of mysticism, was the answer.

Did Dolores substitute mysticism for life? Or did mysticism make life possible, add to life? I think both. Dolores would not have survived without it. She would have disintegrated or society would have crushed her. Mysticism fortified her within and without. It held her together and enabled her to come through repeated periods of disintegration. And it gave her a base or center from which to meet reality on her own terms.

Perhaps she dismissed or discounted huge portions of reality. But she tended to maintain enough of a therapy practice to survive, and had enough points of contact with other liminal souls to make life worthwhile. She would always live from the soul. The conventional mainstream was outside her domain. She was on another track, a mystical substream, a point in the diamond that made fractures glow.

I never felt my job was to make Dolores into a different person, to make her more "realistic." She would never have stayed with a reality-oriented therapist. I was willing to accept that what most people called reality would be meaningless to her. Mystical reality was her home, her world. What was most important was that she make the most of the home and world she lived in.

For an individual like Dolores, growth within the mystical domain is more important than growth outside it. It would be harsh and unrealistic to oppose mystical radiance with practical criticism. One needs to grow along one's own track, not switch to someone else's. One needs to become the sort of person through whom mystical experience can evolve, and who can evolve through mystical experience.

Mystical Maturation

What is important is not mysticism versus other domains, but lack of growth within the mystical domain itself. With a Dolores therapy cannot focus on the domains her brand of mysticism leaves out (mainstream social life, marriage, vocational ambition, economic security or greed). But one can focus on ways her use of mystical experience short-circuits itself.

As a young woman, Dolores became dependent on mystical feeling to offset dread of disintegration. She fell through a trapdoor in her psyche into a world of heightened sensation-feeling that made her feel more whole. The affect of moment was everything. Nothing outside it mattered. In this context, disintegration was part of the cycle of affects, part of a death-rebirth process. Dolores spontaneously found a way to counter disintegrating and going under. Her brand of mystical intensity saved her from madness and death.

Nevertheless, I think it would be wrong to view her mysticism as merely defensive. It tapped into and opened a deeply meaningful reality, perhaps an underpinning or counter-reality to the ticking off of conventional life. She lived in timeless time, a world in which the experience of the moment was real, a world of the realness of experience as such, especially the sensation-feeling side of things.

The sensation-feeling world saved her life. She would be loyal to it forever. She dreaded the intellect's destructive potential, its role as killer of life. Her mother's emphasis on mental superiority contributed to the disintegration she underwent. She knew her mother's pride in mind was wrong. She experienced its destructiveness firsthand. It did not work for her. For Dolores intellect was useful if it enhanced sensation-feeling and cleared the way for more intense states.

Now she had to face the fact that the capacity that opened and saved her (safety net and treasure) kept her from growing. The experiential capacity that enlarged her made her small. She never had been in a position to think of the addictive, tyrannical aspects of mystical states, the slavery, as well as freedom, of mystical moments. These moments had meant too much to be placed in doubt.

It was more than simply finding her mother's self-righteousness buried in the heart of what she valued. This was hard enough. But the matter went beyond maternal infiltration of her deep self. Through our encounter, Dolores discovered for herself the double-edged sense of "rightness" that organizes experience. Her mother's oblivious self-righteousness was damaging. But in the end, we all have to deal with the damage and benefits our sense of rightness brings.

Dolores got a first-hand glimpse of what in literature and religion has variously been described as hubris, original sin, pride, vanity, narcissism, folly, madness, egocentricity, selfishness. The repeated wound to our close tie led to a moment of revisualization of who we were. The hidden "me right—you wrong" sensation that permeated experience was exposed in a way that took Dolores by surprise. Her mother was a damaging carrier of the psychobiological virus, but not its originator. Dolores had no one to blame for the astonishing egocentricity that pervades experience. Her mother's (or my own) horribleness did not make Dolores pure.

Mystical feeling expanded to include two people who could be right *and* wrong, and for whom terms like *right* and *wrong* are crude or beside the point (unless one wants to spend one's life arguing). The mystical glow expanded to include two people fighting for their lives, finding and losing each other, combatants, friends, partners, loved ones, ready to be touched by what it is possible to go through together, ready to try again.

The glow of self expanded to include glowing selves in various states of realization. We were touched by each other through all the breaks between us. It was as if we were saying that there is a goodness in life that runs deeper than the ghastly things that happen. We were uplifted by the regeneration of this goodness, repeated miracles of refinding each other.

For someone like Dolores, who must progress within a mystical field, therapy enlarges the area of intersubjective glow or numinosity or charge, so that it includes perceived shifts in two subjects, variably closer-further from each other, in ways that neither subject can finally destroy or decisively warp. The mystical field expanded to include the possibility of a faulty relationship regenerating at deep levels. The torn heart became part of a larger flow.

We were developing a relationship that made room for changes Dolores went through alone. Not only could we go through them together, we could go through much more, much else. The possibility of what two people could endure and survive together was incessantly redefined. Difficulties that would have led to breakdowns of relationships became challenges for growth. We tasted what it was like to be inspired by going through places there seemed no way out of. The gates of hell could not stop us. We kept coming back for more.

This is like and unlike what Dolores has gone through in her life. Yes, her mother will always love her, accept her. But her mother does not know her, has not found her, hasn't the slightest idea who she is. The repair therapy offers involves seeing, feeling, being in ways a person can say, Yes, this is me, this is more like it, a place I want more of. We discover that our relationship survives us, and we survive it. We are resources for our relationship, and it for us. We learn to take into account how destructive we can be, and survive this learning.

Rebirth remains central, but takes on a different quality. It is not simply the shift from low to high or breaking through a wall that counts. There is also a sense of self-other generating and regenerating each other in many keys, always another corner to be turned. Peak intensity combines with openness to time, as notes in a phrase, parts of an ever-changing song we never get enough of. We bob up and find each other just as we thought we would be alone forever. But now we know that finding is possible, that we never stop making each other possible.

PRECOCIOUS MALEVOLENCE-BENEVOLENCE, PRECOCIOUS AFFECT, UNBORN TOGETHER, NEW CONNECTIONS

Dolores was one of the least hurtful persons I've ever met. She could become furiously enraged when she felt violated. But I never felt injured by her. This is in contrast to individuals who chronically injure others, whose very being seems to be injurious. One can't get near such people without getting bloody.

Charles Manson is an extreme example of precocious mystical malevolence that forecloses flow of experience. More generally, devil cults twist experience out of shape, and glory in hate. One cannot penetrate the veil of self-justificatory "rightness" that grips fanatics. The malevolent mystic cannot bear the Other's claim to goodness or creativeness. He prefers a counterworld of his making to the world's injustices. In a way, he is like Dolores, before she saw she could be wrong. Dolores, however, does not injure or kill anyone by shrinking (expanding) her world to mystical moments (although her mother may be baffled, disappointed, chagrined). The malevolent mystic requires elimination of target others, or parts of others. He cannot rest until some other is injured or disposed of. If looks could kill, his job would be easier. But he usually must go through the trouble of developing or finding means to implement his evil vision. He may become a magnet for others who crave violent "solutions" for complex tensions.

Certain kinds of love also foreclose flow of experience. Maternal love that upholds her child's being may violate the latter's person. A mother may forever picture her child as younger and other than he is. Her vision of the child's goodness may be maddening, insofar as she does not have an inkling of the tormented soul he really is. The child may desperately up the ante until someone responds to his grief. Individuals use various affect patterns to simplify experience and harden or soften personality enough to excite (or dismiss) attention and to function.

Affect, not only intellect, may be precociously organized. We become specialists in certain affects and their patternings as ways of giving ourselves identities, feeling real, or avoiding unspeakable horrors. Dolores discovered she could use intense affect moments to develop a way of life. As long as she knew she could dip into moments of heightened affect, she would be all right. Other people functioned as stimuli for heightened states, and, to some extent, as mood modifiers. This worked well enough, until her sensitivity threatened to swallow her, perhaps swallow itself as well.

Our mystical sensitivities hooked into each other. We jostled for position before relaxing into deeper currents. We tugged at each other. Who would lead where? The idea of leader faded. We shifted positions like birds in flight, fish in water, animate, sensitive, molecular waves.

Dolores's imaginative life more readily embraced the play of sensations, feelings, and thoughts. The gap between sophisticated ideals and embryonic realities was mitigated by the pleasure Dolores and I got by being unborn together. We blanked out and grew from our points of pain many times. We went through nothing and through hell so often, and in so many ways, that faith in our radiant connection deepened. Mystical appreciation of being no longer short-circuited growth of personality, but became integral to it.

For Dolores and myself, personal growth was inherently mystical, and mystical awareness became allied with personal growth. This involved a realignment and reworking of the connection between the capacity for mystical experience and the capacity for personality growth. Our relationship became a place where capacities that did not necessarily work together had a chance to link up in new ways.

In Dolores's life, mystical awareness and personality growth fed each other up to a point. But they would become incendiary, warring parties, forcing Dolores to pull back, shrink. Mystical feelings often jettisoned Dolores's growth. The mystical capacity could become parasitic, feeding off Dolores's personality, rather than feeding it. At such moments, Dolores would be terrified of her personality and mystical capacity. Our relationship shifted the psychospiritual balance for the better, since it was allied both with mystical awareness and personal growth. There are people who fear psychotherapy will be destructive to their mystical selves, and people who fear mysticism will be destructive to their personal selves. There are many individuals, like Dolores, who cannot feel real without working out ways for these capacities to feed each other.

SUMMARY

It is important to recognize that capacities that save an individual may also thwart her. Dolores lucked out by stumbling on a sort of sensory-soul mystical sensitivity that made life meaningful and intense. At the same time, her sensitivity threatened to swallow her up and stifle growth. Her intense tie to her therapist unmasked a hidden omniscience or tyrannical sense of rightness parasitically embedded in mystical feeling. Buried at the heart of her ideology of openness was, ironically, a moralistic and judgmental element that made life unbearable. It made her openness rigid and brittle so that she felt on the edge of breakdown.

The missing hate in her life gnawed at her from within. Mystical feeling provided a home for the megalomanic inflation pervading the parental objects that nurtured-attacked-debased her. Primary objects provided her with an atmosphere of poisonous nurture that she tried to transcend. Therapy provided an object she could fight and fuse with, one who valued mystical communion and personal growth. Neither Dolores nor I had to camouflage our desire for everything in abject, spineless maneuvers in any final way. Very often the miserable states we got ourselves into turned out to be fun. In time, we could count on coming through ourselves together.

REFERENCES

Bion, W. R. (1965). *Transformations*. London: Heinemann.
—— (1967). *Second Thoughts*. New York: Jason Aronson, 1983.
Eigen, M. (1992). *Coming Through the Whirlwind*. Wilmette, IL; Chiron.
Lacan, J. (1777). *Ecrits*. New York: W. W. Norton.
—— (1978). *The Four Fundamental Concepts of Psycho-Analysis*. New York: W. W. Norton.
Rodman, R. F. (1987). *The Spontaneous Gesture: Selected Letters of D. W. Winnicott*. Cambridge: Harvard University Press.
Winnicott, D. W. (1958). *Collected Papers–Through Paediatrics to Psycho-Analysis*. New York: Basic Books.
—— (1965). *The Maturational Processes and the Facilitating Environment*. New York: International Universities Press.
—— (1971). *Playing and Reality*. New York: Basic Books.
—— (1974). Fear of breakdown. *International Review of Psycho-Analysis* 1:103–107.

7

Cannibalization of the Self: Children of the Inner City

Ira J. Schaer
Raymond J. Vasser

Premature ego development has generally focused on precocious verbal or ideational abilities, from Freud's (1913) speculations about the pathogenesis of obsessional neurosis to James's (1960) and Kelly's (1970) exploration of this phenomenon in clinical work with children. Later writings have delineated the emotional costs to the personality, such as Kulish's (1988) description of the early disappointment in the parental object that the child is compelled to recognize, resulting in a premature sense of autonomy and disillusionment in and deflation of the parental imago. Little has been said about precocious motor development or hypercathexis of the sensory-perceptual system—ego functions in conjunction with their related ego apparatuses that could potentially be placed under control of the infant at a very early time. While rarely included in the typography of precocious development, which is usually meant to include such sophisticated refinements as highly advanced musical, artistic, or intellectual skills, a group of capabilities known in the vernacular as "street smarts" might well assume this mantle when viewed from a very different cultural perspective. Our work with chronically abused inner-city children affords the opportunity to explore an altogether different form of precocious development, a precocity that ultimately cripples and cannibalizes the self that it initially strove to preserve.

Children of the inner cities, the most violent, crime-ridden, and poverty-stricken areas of the United States, have little choice other than to adapt to their environment. Whether they find themselves the victimized or the victimizers, or both, they must traverse a dangerous course that rarely affords second chances. From earliest infancy, they are schooled in how to survive, in how to "talk the talk" and "walk the walk." They develop an array of survival skills that allows them to negotiate their streets and neighborhoods with a minimal risk of harm, although they quickly learn the first rule: there are no guarantees. A sense of fatalism and magical thinking comes to mute the anxiety attendant on realizing that life sometimes really is a crapshoot, that little is predictable or constant other than eruptive, erratic violence, as in that of a drive-by shooting.

The children we see have an interesting combination of skills and deficits; their commonality lies in respective histories of documented chronic physical and sexual abuse, deprivation, and neglect. Utilizing Freud's (1920) most restrictive definition of trauma, it is an excitation powerful enough to break through the stimulus barrier and consequently flood the ego with stimulation that it can neither bind to nor dispose of; these children are indeed traumatized, and chronically so. Freud (1926) stated it explicitly:

> In relation to the traumatic situation, in which the subject is helpless, external and internal dangers, real dangers and instinctual demands converge. Whether the ego is suffering from a pain which will not stop or experiencing an accumulation of instinctual needs which cannot obtain satisfaction, the economic situation is the same, and the motor helplessness of the ego finds expression in psychical helplessness. [p. 168]

The ego is designated as the central victim in a traumatic event. From the outset, an important component of the concept of trauma has been its central victim, the ego, and the ego is most susceptible to damage in infancy (A. Freud 1967). Winnicott (1989) also linked the notion of trauma with the age of onset, as well as the concept of impingement: "Trauma is an impingement from the environment and from the individual's reaction to the environment that occurs prior to the individual's development of the mechanisms that make the unpredictable predictable" (p. 198). Lacking ego support or protection from the holding environment, the mother, the infant is compelled to "react" rather than respond, interrupting the infant's "going on being" and threatening mental stability.

Thus, the ego is rendered helpless, or traumatized, by virtue of a failure of the mother to hold the infant and protect it from being impinged upon. Faced with these impingements or overwhelming anxieties, the infant is compelled to develop certain skills or capacities that enable it to survive. James (1960) went so far as to speculate that if a profound failure of mothering occurred within the first few months of life, hypercathexis of specific mental apparatus would result, leading to a physiological organ compliance or facilitation at both a physical as well as a psychological level. The infant is compelled to accommodate him- or herself to the mother by virtue of survival. With many inner-city children, a characteristic pattern evolves between mother and child that has been referred to as "working for the mother," where the mother remains narcissistically invested in her infant only as long as the infant gratifies her. The mother overgratifies the infant out of her own sense of personal deprivation, inevitably withdrawing her supplies as she becomes increasingly jealous that the infant is "getting what I never got." Inescapably the mother turns from indulgence to deprivation, claiming to do otherwise would risk "spoiling" her 3-week-old.

Reacting first to mother's cold, physical withdrawal with its threatened loss of emotional and physical sustenance, the infant is compelled to be hypervigilant to her cues, reacting to mother's needs for gratification so she will respond to him. A precocious reactivity to the environment develops, with a concomitant narcissistic identification with aspects of the mother beginning to form. In contrast to a more typical situation where mother remains exquisitely sensitive and responds to her infant's cues, here the mother responds only to those aspects of her baby's behavior that unconsciously meet her demands to be mothered and gratified by the infant. Hendrick (1951) speaks of an analogous process that involves an early ego identification with partial ego functions of the mother. Khan (1963) explicates a selective ego development of emergent ego functions that are exploited for self-defense and survival. This hypervigilance to mother and the premature narcissistic identification with her partial ego functions and needs for gratification are the very essence of reacting to an environmental impingement that Winnicott describes; this hypervigilance represents a precocious ego development.

The hypercathexis of the sensory-perceptual system is only a part of the precocity compelled by the "working for the mother." Kelly (1970) notes that motility is available at an early age for acceleration of ego functions. The environment can selectively reinforce the development of gross and fine motor discharge channels by taking particular pleasure in a child's motor skills, viewing them as a sign of early intelligence, athletic potential, and sexual prowess, and heralding the beginning of a parentally less-demanding toddlerhood. The mother's failure to be available compels the infant not only to seduce or coerce mother's participation, but also to fall back on its own motoric capacities to regulate homeostasis by ridding itself of excess, noxious internal or external stimulation through motoric discharge. By selective, narcissistic reinforcement of motoric displays and the infant's precocious self-reliance on its motoric system to discharge large quantums of noxious stimulation, the motor-discharge system becomes increasingly cathected and overutilized.

Many of these children have been subject throughout their lives to chronic, unremitting physical and sexual abuse, as well as deprivation and neglect. Winnicott (1975) believed that impingements that demanded excessive reactions could not be contained by the infant through the premature utilization of the mind as a substitute for primary maternal preoccupation. He speculated that either confusion would result or that the reactions to these impingements would be catalogued through a process he referred to as "exact memorizing." He illustrated this point by describing impingements during the birth process in which there was a severe disturbance of continuity resulting in this exact memorizing. Winnicott believed that this cataloging will remain fixed because it occurred early enough in development that the psyche-soma was unable to dispose of it.

Birth trauma aside, many of these children do come into the world in a highly distressed state (e.g., cocaine/crack addicted, low birth weight, premature) for which even the most perfect of mothers would have difficulty compensating. The sad reality is that many of these mothers are children themselves with severe problems in terms of their own narcissism and paucity of environmental support. During the period of earliest infancy these children are subjected to significant environmental impingements that occur prior to a time that the psyche-soma is sophisticated enough to deal with them, concomitant with a failure of the mothering object to adequately hold the infant. An exact memorizing of the environmental impingements may occur, which is etched at a sensorimotor level due to the primitive state of the organism. This may well become the analog for the sensorimotor reenactments that we so often see with these children, a kind of cataloging of the early traumatic impingements through motoric acting out. This is only compounded by the child's later need to resort to a reenactment as a reflection, if not a direct communication, of their internal state of being overwhelmed.

This precocious motor skill development reverberates throughout ego growth, specifically in terms of an acquired overreliance on these channels to discharge accumulated tension, often to the neglect or detriment of more highly advanced and efficient mechanisms. Greenacre (1967) notes that actual trauma leaves an organized imprint in the ego, patterning the discharge of all impulses while encouraging repetition through action. In this way the ego becomes channelized, with a propensity to discharge any tension immediately. Any frustrating event that might otherwise become nutriment for ego enhancement largely escapes the control of higher-level ego functioning. Thus, cognitive and later abstract reasoning abilities are interfered with, symbol formation and language development are truncated. Ultimately, there is a failure to use fantasy to work through conflicts, the child remains stimulus bound and concrete, tending to use action or action language rather than mental representation.

The combination of sensory-perceptual and motor skill overreliance, originally initiated to remain hyperalert to mother's presence and needs, progressively shapes the ego while accommodating itself to reality; these hypertrophied functions later emerge as survival skills. Thus these children become "street smart" at an early age, able to spot trouble or a potentially dangerous situation rapidly with an uncanny ability to read adults and situations. They live in a realistically dangerous world that is often unpredictable and frightening; by their elementary school years they are able to negotiate and thrive in a hostile environment.

The hypertrophy of sensorimotor channels is not the only problematic development. Precocity also leads to the development of a highly elaborated false-self system. Winnicott (1965) described the false self, stating that a mother who failed to meet her infant's gesture could instead substitute her own gesture, thus compelling her infant to comply with her needs. The infant's compliance is the earliest stage of the false self, indicating the mother's inability to sense her infant's needs. Through utilizing the false self, the child builds up a false set of relationships to itself and others. Winnicott linked this development to a need to re-create or evoke further impingements to the personality: "Instead of cultural pursuits one observes in such people extreme restlessness, an inability to concentrate, and a need to collect impingements from external reality so that the living time of the individual can be filled by reactions to these impingements" (p. 150).

We see an infant who, if it is to be mothered by its own mother, must respond and remain hypersensitive to mother's unconscious, narcissistic needs, selectively identifying with mother's needs while mothering the mother. Ultimately, the child must give up its own self-differentiation to work for the mother, taking on her attributes or mothering functions in contrast to establishing its own unique differentiated identity. The character becomes one based on narcissistic identifications and attributes, with anxiety over abandonment by the mother allayed by a joining or merger with the mothering object (Kelly 1970, Khan 1963, Kulish 1988). Disappointment with the mother turns to disillusionment and then rage, as erratic swings of overwhelming gratification turn to either neglect or deprivation. Not infrequently, the swing does not stop there but proceeds full circle to physical abuse and assault, the mother becoming increasingly enraged as she must give to her child what she felt she never got or deserved. Initially overidentifying with her infant's helplessness, she now becomes her own powerful mother by identifying with the aggressor.

The infant and the young child are compelled to meld two contradictory if not antithetical views of the maternal object together, a task beyond the skills of an adult with a fully functioning defensive armamentarium. The child is compelled to vertically split the object, completely ablating the "bad" part of the object, and melded with it that part of the "bad" self, preserving only the "good" part object and the complementary part of the "good" self. This is the process described by Shengold (1989) in his description of "soul murder." Krystal (1978) describes another part of the process where the child splits off experience from affect and eventually affect from memory. Memory itself becomes threatening and looming, bringing with it fears of further disappointment and rage. Acting out or reenactment can serve as a defense against remembering in words or thought, acting to obliterate the affects associated with the painful memories.

The exact memorizing with its propensity to forward the development of precocious motor skills and the compelled hypervigilance to the mother lay the groundwork for the street smarts so vital for survival in this dangerous environment. The creation of the false self in response to the massive impingements drains liveliness away from the infant and child, leaving a hollow sense of self and fragmented relatedness to others. In response to repeated deprivations, neglect, and erratic mothering, a smoldering sense of bitterness is generated that transforms unrequited dependency needs into a predatory stance toward their world—a sense of hardened entitlement. Thus the self is cannibalized to ensure the individual's survival.

However, this situation may only speak to the infant or child of "average endowment" faced with the prototypical impingements of inner-city life. There are a gifted few who seem not only to survive but to flourish on these mean streets. These are the children with street smarts or skills in reading and negotiating their way in the ghetto that surpass even their peers' uncanny ability to sniff out danger before it happens or to be able to size up others in terms of their potential danger or exploitability. These are the "players" who learn quickly how to manipulate others, to "score," whether in terms of economic gain or aggressive and/or sexual prowess. They have a highly developed verbal facility used either for presentation of self (e.g., rapping) or as part of an action (e.g., running a con), often gaining much admiration and status from peers. This is, above all, a culturally syntonic and recognized way of beating the system, more often than not without direct redress to physical violence.

What of the child of exceptional mental endowment who is paired with a mother who possesses far more nurturant capabilities but is still victimized by her physical and psychological circumstances? A mother who may be chronically depressed or overwhelmed, but who does provide for her child in an albeit erratic fashion? It is under these circumstances that we anticipate that the infant will be compelled to replace the mother with his mind, to embrace his mind as the very center of his liveliness and to provide for himself the self-care and self-holding that the environment will not relinquish. This brings us to the acquaintance of a remarkable little boy who compelled us to rethink our conceptualizations of development in the inner city.

CASE STUDY

Tony, a 7-year-old African-American child, demonstrates several behavioral and clinical manifestations that represent the special brand of precocity seen in some inner-city children. Although he presented himself as capable from the outset, he was truly masterful at concealing his deep insecurities and a prevailing sense of emptiness and rage. Geared for survival, he had developed rather enviable street smarts, but he would ultimately pay a steep price for his highly burnished bravado. At times he acted like a sensory processing machine, sizing up a situation in a moment and reacting. Reading the moods of others, he could prepare to defend himself if he detected anger. Conversely, he would pursue a self-serving manipulation with engaging charm and wit if he detected a pliable, friendly audience. It was only after many hours that the veneer of his omnipotence and his advanced capabilities wore through revealing the stark, encapsulated world of the mind object.

During the initial evaluation, prior to his admission to the inpatient unit of the children's service of the Detroit Psychiatric Institute, his mother reported an extensive history of behavioral problems including frequent fights, explosive temper tantrums, incorrigibility and a long history of setting fires since he was 3 years old. When Tony set his mother's mattress on fire and nearly destroyed their apartment building, she feared for her own and her daughter's safety.

Tony was the second of two children born to a 15-year-old single mother. Ms. G. stated that she was unaware of the pregnancy until she was 18 to 20 weeks pregnant. While there were no reports of any medical difficulties prenatally or at birth, by 6 weeks Tony was diagnosed as having bronchial asthma. Early home life was punctuated by chronic, explosive violence and episodic neglect. Shortly after Tony's birth, he and his mother moved in with his maternal aunt whose boyfriend was assaultive and suspected of abusing the children. Tony's father occasionally stopped by, but these visits frequently degenerated into drug-induced tirades targeting Tony and his mother. Episodes of physical abuse, "whoopings," were typically employed to discipline the children. Drug abuse was common among the residents of the home, and the children consequently were frequently unsupervised and neglected. They observed repeated instances of eruptive violence that the adults visited upon themselves, or often found themselves the targets of this violence. Upon Tony's admission to the hospital his mother appeared depressed, dependent, and overwhelmed. The father was antisocial, angry, and hostile.

"Man" was the nickname mother gave her son since he was a toddler. This was not without good reason. To illustrate her point, Ms. G. told of Tony dressing himself up in a sport coat from the age of 5 and leaving the home every Sunday morning for several hours. Tony's mother went on to say that it was just prior to the evaluation that she learned that he was attending services at a church two blocks away in a congregation she had never belonged or even visited. To her amusement, she found that her son had befriended several adult members of this congregation.

When the therapist (Raymond Vasser) first met Tony on the ward, he was immediately struck by this child's demeanor and size, so much so that he seriously doubted that he was talking to the right child. Tony's physical appearance was that of a 10- or 11-year-old (later inquiry revealed that he placed in the 99th percentile for both height and weight for 9-year-old boys; for a 7-year-old, he was completely off the scale). A handsome, dark-complected youngster who extended his hand for a firm handshake when first introduced, he maintained good eye contact as he was informed that he would meet for therapy the following Monday. He responded by asking the purpose of this meeting, cautioning that he did not yet know his schedule. Tony advised the therapist that he should check with the ward staff whether Tony would be available at the time of the appointment, as he anticipated that school might conflict with the appointment time. He was assured that the therapist would work with the staff to coordinate meetings with the ward schedule.

Tony managed his first session with the same degree of aplomb noted in our first encounter. Openly stating that he was "glad" to be in the hospital, he then confided that he had learned more both about the ward schedule and about some of the children on the ward. He knew that each child met with a therapist several times per week and wondered if his therapist knew a particular boy who had a reputation for acting out. This discussion occurred seamlessly as he slowly investigated the office and its contents.

Strikingly absent were any concerns of being separated from his family; instead he was confident and curious. Indeed he was so confident and evidently at ease with the situation that one had the uncanny impression that this young boy fancied himself as having just arrived at some exclusive spa and was now quite naturally in his "element." Volunteering rather blandly that he was in the hospital solely because his sister "said" that he had set a mattress on fire, he denied any responsibility, adding almost as a stage aside that his sister was well known to lie about the facts. Well prepared to plead his case, he never admitted the least bit of guilt. He did allow, grudgingly, that his real problem was his sister who chronically tried to make him look bad.

Curious about the structure of the therapy sessions, he pressed the therapist to tell him how long they would meet and whether he would miss school to attend the sessions. While charming and engaging, he seemed driven to size up the situation and to quickly learn the ground rules. Most impressive was his assured, confident manner—much more like a confident teenager than a 7-year-old boy.

As the treatment progressed, Tony would anticipate scheduling problems, often volunteering possible options for rescheduling, or in a more philosophical mood offering suggestions for improvements on the ward. Upon learning that children occasionally went home for the weekend on the recommendation of the treatment team, he inquired as to who was on the team. This was merely a preface to his real question as to why he was not a team member. A year later, as an outpatient, he would ride two buses through Detroit for his therapy sessions, as his sister or mother was often unable to accompany him. He largely took personal responsibility for calling to make, cancel, or reschedule appointments.

Tony's blend of savoir faire, humor, and the ability to read people served him nicely. The ward staff, teachers, and clinical staff all liked him. Engaging and self-assured, he seemed satisfied in a world of his own construction. He never seemed to rely on others, preferring instead to find his own way in spite of whatever obstacles he encountered. What appeared of utmost importance was to disavow his attachment to others. He was in his element running "cons" or "scams" on others, but it was terrifying for him to admit any feelings of dependency through a display of ignorance, feelings of affection, attachment, or need. As a consequence, schoolwork suffered as he found it difficult to subordinate himself to the rank of student, preferring instead to teach rather than be taught.

Soon Tony learned the limits placed on his wishes to explore the office. His questions about the therapist and his wishes to investigate the desk, personal locker, and file cabinet were frustrated. He revealed fantasies that the therapist possessed unlimited supplies of food, primarily treats and "goodies." He considered the locker and desk the repositories of the best treats. Feeling excluded and discounted, at first he cajoled and tried to seduce with flattery but this soon gave way to insistence and threats. A particularly striking vignette from the early sessions illustrates this:

> Tony entered the office and smelled that I had tea earlier in the day. He went to the trash can to find the evidence of my rebuff. Finding the spent tea bag, he chastised me for not

sharing with him. While rummaging through the trash he casually announced: "I bet you didn't know I was a garbage picker." He then produced a Ziploc bag.

Partially filling the bag with water from the sink, he held the bag to his breast while parading about the office asking how well I like him and his "titty." After biting a small hole in the bag, he was able to squirt a small stream of water by squeezing the bag. He the held the bag to his breast while alternately walking around swinging his hips and squirting water into his mouth.

Directing my intervention to the grandiose defense of his self-reliance, I observed: "Yes, Tony, it would be nice not to have to rely on anyone else for those things that you really need. Then you wouldn't have to feel so scared and hurt when you do not or cannot get what you want, like tea or like things that you find as 'off limits' in the office." In response, he placed the bag to his crotch and squirted the office and me. I offered; "Even my saying so brings out your angry feelings about being left out. Those feelings are so strong that you want to piss on me and everything else."

Illustrated here are Tony's fragile, narcissistic vulnerability, seeking love equivalents in the form of oral supplies, and qualitative aspects of internalized representations of himself and others. He provided us with a glimpse of what would later crystallize into an enduring transference, while exposing the roots of both his precocity and his destructive rage.

This is just one demonstration of Tony's heightened sensory attunement. He was hyperalert and hypersensitive to the point of being able to detect the presence of an unopened box of tea inside a locked desk drawer. The spent tea bag at the bottom of the trash can was sufficient stimulus for a search. Convinced that once again he has been deprived and neglected, redress and triumph were attained by locating evidence of my crime. His offhand reference to himself as a "garbage picker" revealed his experience of self as one who must settle for discarded scraps, a striking contrast to the cool, self-assured, and omnipotent man-child who could scam adults and hold his own on the streets.

His disappointment was kept at bay as he prepared his own "drink." Demonstrating his resourceful ability to provide for himself, he thus denied any need for others by creating his own breast. More than a passing reference to his relationship with his mother, it was a fundamental enactment of his own experience of himself with others. He might settle for water now, but he knew there was tea and milk somewhere out there. His provocatively swinging hips were a seduction to the therapist into loving him or at the very least into gratifying him. The therapist's intervention was intended to tap into the rageful side of his disappointment at being neglected, while confronting him with his characterological defense of becoming grandiose and omnipotent in the face of his felt helplessness and neediness.

This vignette also illuminates the darker, more troubling aspects of Tony's inner world. The essential theme was to be repeated countless times in the course of the work. In the transference he continued to re-create and reenact the utterly disappointing elements of his relationship with his mother, and his attempts to extract from the outside what he felt he had been deprived of. Cast into the role of the depriving, self-absorbed, and self-serving mother, the therapist was seen to withhold all that which promised Tony internal pleasure or comfort. He associated what he could cajole, seduce, con, or steal as prized trophies of either his streetwise self-sufficiency or his lovableness. Constantly frustrated, he abandoned his pursuits toward the therapist as the other and turned instead to his own devices. If the therapist failed to give up what he needed, he made it quite clear that he was well equipped to take it back by force or subterfuge. He spent long periods of time trying to pick the locks on the drawers and locker. He would frequently attempt to race into the kitchen where he would grab handfuls of sugar, smiling broadly when the therapist arrived moments later to direct him back to the office.

His turning away from the therapist in the transference appeared to duplicate his experience of the early disruption of his narcissistic orbit. It appeared that Tony's early attempts to please his mother became a one-sided, frustrating appeal, predisposing him to turn instead either to manipulating the environment to gain control of a frightening, empty internal and external world or instead to identifying with aspects of her mothering and trying to mother her to seduce her compliance. Failing in this, he ultimately turned inward and overvalued his abilities to coerce from the environment what it refused to give him. Stealing the precious supplies thus became poetic justice to those who had so basely stolen or withheld from him.

Unable or at times unwilling to look inside, he was constantly focused on those around him, scanning them to rapidly ascertain their likes and dislikes. When he found a chessboard in the office, he inquired about the rules and, with the help of other children and the ward staff, mastered the basic openings and moves in less than two weeks. Tony was intensely curious about the therapist, his car, and his home life. He pretended that he had met the therapist's wife, informing him that he found her to be "as pretty as Whitney Houston," easily understanding why the therapist had married her.

In early sessions he expressed the wish to be white, like his therapist, emerging from the lavatory with his face covered in a creamy, white lather of soap. He used brown, black, and gray markers to draw a beard onto his face and scissors to cut hair from the top of his head, attempting to mirror the therapist's appearance. The therapist was taken aback by other behaviors that were clearly an accurate reflection of his mannerisms. Taking his desk chair, Tony would lean back, cross his legs, hold his chin and ask the therapist to tell him (Tony) "what feelings or ideas" he had about a particular issue. The therapist had to admit to some discomfort as it appeared as if he were staring into a mirror, so accurate was Tony's impersonation.

Most remarkable was his ability to adopt more subtle attributes of the therapist's personality. After a particularly difficult session during which Tony needed to be physically restrained for most of the thirty minutes, he asked me, "Where did you get those asshole shoes? Probably at the asshole shoe store, on the asshole street where assholes like you live." I tied his behavior to angry feelings that maybe he doesn't even know about; I told him it is those feelings and worries that we must understand. Settled, he offered me a suggestion: "You know, Mr. Vasser, if you went to the Footlocker you could get some other shoes, like Reeboks, and then you would be cool." The humor of the moment struck me, and I commented, "With all the exercise we've been getting in here lately, perhaps it's a good idea that I get some athletic shoes." Surprised, he turned to me and laughed.

Looking back, it was obvious that Tony had several reactions to the therapist's intervention. Of those, his most important response was to the self-disclosure implied in the therapist's offhand comment. Upon reflection, it did not surprise the therapist that he would have offered such a response as a way to titrate his own feelings of frustration and anger, as well as physical fatigue. Tony appeared to have some intuitive knowledge of that purpose, and the therapist found himself again looking into the same mirror when Tony would use wit tinged with cynicism as a buffer to some of his own turbulent feelings.

In another session, Tony composed and choreographed an impromptu rap about how tough, mean, and bad he was. I responded with my own "interpretive rap" gently confronting his defense of invulnerability by saying, "I know this lad who thinks he's bad, he tries to be tough so he'll never feel sad." There was a long, theatrical pause as he gaped at me with a look of hopeless disbelief. He slowly lowered his chin, looking at me as if over the top of his imaginary glasses, and said, "Do you call that a rap?"

This vignette and many similar ones helped to explain Tony's engaging demeanor and why people liked him. His finely honed capacity to imitate others was often rather flattering to the person that he imitated. Additionally, Tony hints at his early experiences where he may have learned that his survival and association with caregivers was contingent upon his ability to both read and perform for others. Speculatively, this might have been the prototypical experience of "working for the mother," maintaining a bond to her through his ability to identify with her while gratifying her own narcissistic needs. The child learns early on to read and respond to others at the expense of his own needs and individuation while struggling with his own emptiness and rage over a life—his own—not lived.

Tony's precocious abilities came at a considerable expense to his development and overall functioning. His need to "operate on" or "con" those around him precluded the opportunity to learn and grow emotionally, or to developmentally establish what Sarnoff (1976) refers to as the "structure of latency." As noted above, he was constantly focused on the therapist during sessions. His focus was driven and compulsive, with Tony rarely playing spontaneously or engaging in play fantasy. The therapist felt that he was under the microscope every moment of the session, with his every action coolly scrutinized and catalogued by Tony. This child was easily flooded by strong feelings, often leading to violent enactments, resisting deeper explorations of his disappointment and rage. Empathic skills were not utilized to draw closer to others, but to charm, manipulate, and control. He appeared fixed in an archaic world of anger and disappointment.

Tony appeared to have little capacity to feel good about himself in the absence of continual praise or repartee. He saw himself as a "garbage picker" whose experiences of abuse and neglect were logical precursors to how worthless he felt. His consequent feelings of helplessness and fear were glossed over by his grandiosity and his ability to charm. Not surprisingly, he found little pleasure in his own accomplishments. Unlike a 5-year-old who shouts "Yes!" to himself in triumphant satisfaction at the completion of a difficult task, Tony could neither complete the task without constant support nor take pleasure in his own accomplishments by looking to others for praise and an affirmation of his own self-value.

Tony illustrates the manifestations of a special brand of precocity seen in some inner-city children. Steeped in a world of violence and neglect, this child's development was distorted for the sake of precocious adaptations that kept him safe and maintained a more or less favorable relationship with his caregivers. We believe Tony to be one such child who's precocious independence, hypervigilance, overvalued ability to manipulate and run "cons" on others, and his capacity to read others were sophisticated expressions of early defensive adaptations. These defenses staved off potential further abuse and a feeling of helplessness by taking his survival skills as his most precious possession. However, his "con" was at the expense of his capacity to develop a more positive sense of himself through usual latency-age channels. He had one "game" that he continually replayed in an elegant but compulsive fashion. His savoir faire, hypervigilance, pseudo-empathy, assuming the attributes of others, and his "conning" all constituted a game he played well, but ultimately at the expense of his overall psychological development.

In retrospect, perhaps one incident that occurred shortly before the formal treatment terminated illuminates the changes that Tony made throughout his therapy. Stomping into the therapist's private office, Tony threw himself on the couch and exclaimed, "I'm so frustrated with my mom and sister!" He then proceeded to go on at length about their evident failures toward him. A seemingly mundane incident in psychotherapy, but not for Tony. He did not act out, he did not trash the room, he did not provocatively reenact with the therapist by having him deprive or frustrate him in something he wanted but well knew he could not have, nor did he pour on the charm and try and manipulate the therapist into gratifying him in some way. He simply verbalized his frustration and tolerated the unpleasant affects that accompanied this rather typical set of deprivations from his family. He was able to trust that the therapist would hear him and help him work through his feelings.

Tony had developed a more serviceable array of defenses at a far greater level of sophistication. His ability to utilize his therapist as a therapist rather than merely as an alternate source of gratification, paired with his growing trust in him, underlay Tony's movement toward genuine relatedness. He could allow the therapist to help him, unmasking dependency wishes that had always been present but were buried defensively behind critical denigration of the other or omnipotently assuming the role of the manipulator or con artist. Tony's long bus ride from Detroit to the suburbs, which involved a number of bus changes and was often undertaken alone, spoke to his recognition and acceptance of his need for the therapist. His wit and humor remained his favored mechanisms to handle disappointment, but the sarcastic, biting edge mellowed a bit. Tony lost none of his precocity or his street sense, although his dreams lost some of their defensive grandiosity as he turned to less glamorous avenues to reach his goals (e.g., getting a job at the car wash at age 12). Along with his capacity to verbalize and think through rather than act out, and his ability to tolerate affect and relatedness with the other, perhaps Tony's greatest achievement rested in his slowly burgeoning capacity for empathy. Tony had come to recognize and turn toward the object world with all of its attendant frustrations, rather than relying on his own mind as his only object.[1]

---

1. After Tony's termination of therapy, the therapist would hear from Tony when he called about once every six months. In early 1992 he called to ask if the therapist would come visit him in the hospital. He stated that he had been shot in a drive-by shooting with serious injuries to both legs. This now 12-year-old boy had secured employment at a car wash and found himself, as he put it, "in the wrong place, at the wrong time!" Two days later the therapist visited him at the hospital and heard all the details of the shooting, his weekend visit to intensive care, several surgeries, and other thankfully less traumatic aspects of his life. When the therapist announced after ninety minutes that he needed to get back to his office, Tony said with a wry smile, "So, you're going to desert me like all the rest?" As a "farewell for now," he encapsulated the entire course and theme of the work with the same wit and charm.

CONCLUSION

This case illustrates one example of those children who possess exceptional endowment yet are nonetheless put at an extreme disadvantage due to the unavailability of the mothering object to act as a reliable and consistent holding environment. Here we find the child relying on his mind, providing for himself the self-care that is not forthcoming from his mother. Consonant with the specific form of precocity seen in his peers, hypervigilance and wariness are elevated to high art forms. Advanced verbal capacities and a keenly developed sense of being able to "read" the other results in a highly sophisticated presentation of the self as street smart or a "player." Perhaps it should come as no surprise that an immense amount of pride is taken in the fact that one can take care of oneself, that one does not need anyone else to support or even care for him. By running the con, the other is made foolish if not completely denigrated, thus further distancing oneself from either one's need or disappointment in the other. The ability to run the con, to know the streets and reliably exploit others, while avoiding entanglements or commitments, becomes the center of the player's liveliness—the embrace of one's own mind as an object.

Anna Freud (1967) warned that the hypertrophy of one ego function over another might create dangers to the individual's psychic economy: fifty years before, Freud (1913) had mused that some degree of precocity of ego development was typical of human nature. It is indeed tragic that what was once confined to describing a particular aspect of neurotic psychopathology has now come to describe, in a mutated and potentially more virulent form, a distinct proportion of our inner-city children.

REFERENCES

Freud, A. (1967). Comments on trauma. In *Psychic Trauma*, ed. S. S. Furst, pp. 235–245. New York: International Universities Press.

Freud, S. (1913). The disposition to obsessional neurosis. *Standard Edition* 12:311–326.

—— (1920). Beyond the pleasure principle. *Standard Edition* 18:3–66.

—— (1926). Inhibitions, symptoms and anxiety. *Standard Edition* 20:77–175.

Greenacre, P. (1967). The influence of infantile trauma on genetic patterns. In *Psychic Trauma*, ed. S. S. Furst, pp. 108–153. New York: International Universities Press.

Hendrick, I. (1951). Early development of the ego: identification in infancy. *Psychoanalytic Quarterly* 20(1):44–61.

James, M. (1960). Premature ego development: some observations on disturbances in the first three months of life. *International Journal of Psycho-Analysis,* 41(4):288–294.

Kelly, K. (1970). A precocious child in analysis. *Psychoanalytic Study of the Child* 25:122–145. New York: International Universities Press.

Khan, M. (1963). The concept of cumulative trauma. *Psychoanalytic Study of the Child* 18:286–306. New York: International Universities Press.

Krystal, H. (1978). Trauma and affect. *Psychoanalytic Study of the Child* 33:81–116. New Haven, CT: Yale University Press.

Kulish, N. (1988). Precocious ego development and obsessive compulsive neurosis. *Journal of the American Academy of Psychoanalysis* 16(2):167–187.

Sarnoff, C. (1976). *Latency.* New York: Jason Aronson.

Shengold, L. (1989). *Soul Murder: The Effects of Childhood Abuse and Deprivation.* New Haven, CT: Yale University Press.

Winnicott, D. W. (1965). Ego distortion in terms of the true and false self. In *The Maturational Processes and the Facilitating Environment.* Toronto: Clarke, Irwin, 1960.

—— (1975). Mind and its relation to the psyche-soma. In *Through Paediatrics to Psychoanalysis*, pp. 243–254. New York: Basic Books.

—— (1989). The concept of clinical regression compared with that of defence organization. In *Psycho-Analytic Explorations*, pp. 193–199. Cambridge, MA: Harvard University Press.

8

No Space for a Baby: Pseudomaturity in an Urban Little Girl[1]

Stephen Seligman
Maria St. John[2]

This chapter describes Dorian, a 3-year-old girl who acted like an older child, both in and out of her psychotherapy sessions. In the face of early and profound traumatic environmental stresses and failures, she relied on social and verbal dexterity and remarkable resilience. These allowed her to construct a superficial personality structure that helped her manage her powerful anxieties but that detached her from real interpersonal contact and her inner world.

Over the first year of Dorian's life, her mother had withdrawn from her, becoming more and more depressed and making a series of increasingly serious and provocative suicide attempts that resulted in almost continuous placement in psychiatric facilities. Her father was practically reliable, if at a minimal level, but he was emotionally bland and unempathic. Instead, he cultivated endurance and stoicism in his daughter, taking her, for example, on walks for hours on extended trips in the mountain backcountry.

1. The authors wish to thank the members of Tuesday Child Psychotherapy Study Group for their helpful comments.
2. Ms. St. John was the therapist in this case. Dr. Seligman was the clinical supervisor.

On the surface, Dorian seemed to be a plucky and congenial toddler and made a bright impression on adults. In her psychotherapy sessions, she played with an apparent sophistication with symbolic and narrative forms that seemed more characteristic of a 5-year-old. But more often than not, her play was detached, unsustained, with frequent and brittle efforts to contain overwhelming anxiety, and outbreaks of disorganization, regression, and breakdowns. She treated both toys and her therapist with omnipotent control.

The following excerpt from her therapist's notes offers a sense of Dorian's complex and uneven presentation:

> First, and for many weeks, the baby doll in the playroom was ignored. When she was finally acknowledged, it was only to be briskly labeled "Happy Baby" by 2-year-old Dorian. This arrangement was interrupted by a brief period of intense, panicky confusion on Dorian's part as to whether the doll was in fact a happy baby or a sad baby. The possibilities prompted episodes of enuresis and were resolved when Dorian decided that the baby doll was a sad baby, and began each session by banishing her to the oven where the doll remained for the duration of the hour. Dorian insisted to the therapist, "She is a sad baby. You don't like her." Although she would play busily and elaborately with other toys, she carefully avoided the doll. Many months into her treatment Dorian reintroduced the doll into the sessions and reopened the problem of its internal states. One day she produced the doll, rocked her roughly in a rocking chair, which banged the wall repeatedly, and then instructed the therapist to do the same. But before the therapist could inquire at all about her instructions, Dorian was absorbed in play with a different set of toys. Within a few minutes she played with three sets of toys, immersing herself in the new play themes each time and directing the therapist's participation with precise and incessant commands. The rocking of the baby doll was not resumed.

Dorian used her substantial personal resources to create a precocious personality structure that helped hold her together and give her some feeling of being in contact in the world. She did so at great psychological cost, but her environment and constitution interacted in such a way that there were few other possibilities. This chapter will examine Dorian's development and treatment in an effort to illuminate the puzzle of how a young child can show such a striking mix of vulnerability and competence, of regression and pseudo-maturity.

DORIAN AND HER PARENTS

Dorian and her parents, Helen and Gary, were referred for infant–parent psychotherapy when she was 22 months old because there was concern about the effects on Dorian of her mother's repeated suicide attempts and subsequent psychiatric hospitalizations and the many attendant shifts in the circumstances of Dorian's care. Infant–parent psychotherapy is a flexible model of intervention with infants and their families that integrates the usual techniques of psychodynamic intervention into the special situation of parents who face multiple difficulties (Fraiberg 1980, Lieberman and Pawl 1993, Seligman 1994). The referral came from the social worker at the inpatient unit of the county hospital, following Helen's multiple hospitalizations and discharges. At the time of the referral Helen was living at a "three-quarter way house" residential treatment facility, and Dorian was cared for by her father, Gary. Gary had become increasingly responsible for Dorian's care as her mother had become more depressed, withdrawn, and impulsively suicidal.

Infant–parent psychotherapy appeared to be indicated because of Dorian's age, along with the extreme nature of the family situation and its impingement on Dorian. However, although infant–parent psychotherapy frequently emphasizes meetings at which parent(s) and infant are simultaneously present, this intervention soon came to include regular individual meetings between Dorian and the therapist. This approach was a response to Dorian's apparent need for and ability to use a direct therapeutic relationship, along with her mother's unreliability as her withdrawal and suicide attempts continued and led to repeated hospitalization. Regular meetings with Dorian proceeded, along with conjoint meetings that included her and her father and/or mother, and meetings with the parents together and individually.

Despite this effort at regularity and comprehensiveness, Dorian's treatment was characterized by incessant interruptions. This reflected the relentlessness of the disruptions in Dorian's life circumstances. Despite such limitations, treatment did proceed for approximately eighteen months. It was finally terminated as the therapy became increasingly diffuse following Helen's long-term placement in a specialized, long-term unit for chronic suicidal patients at a state hospital at some distance from our clinic, and Gary and Dorian's move to a moderately distant suburb.

History and Background

Helen's childhood was turbulent and traumatic. Her father abandoned the family when she was 2 and her mother was frequently physically absent, emotionally rejecting, and often drunk. Helen was subjected to a variety of traumata, including fraternal and possibly maternal sexual abuse. She abused drugs and was raped by various boys during her adolescence.

When Dorian was born, Helen was 17 years old. Helen became increasingly depressed over the course of Dorian's first year, resigning from more and more of Dorian's care until she would respond to any request from the young toddler with the directive, "Go to Papa."

Helen was hospitalized thirteen times during the first two years of Dorian's life, usually in connection with burning or cutting her wrists and inner arms with razor blades and sometimes consuming large amounts of medication. A pattern of withdrawal and aggressive self-destructiveness was punctuated by occasional moments of emotional availability. Helen would remain silent for long periods, only shrugging her shoulders in response to questions, with her long hair almost entirely hiding her face. At other times, she would be agitatedly distractable. In these states she would smoke almost continuously, wearing a Harley Davidson T-shirt and having a body part pierced if she received permission to leave the program site. There were occasional windows of engaged and reflective sorrow that kept some treatment providers interested, but they would eventually become exasperated with Helen.

Helen and Dorian

Similar patterns characterized Helen's relationship with Dorian, along with a more special, if desperate and narcissistically self-serving, mode of relating: Helen would engulf Dorian in a routine of intimate mutual admiration. Often she would take the toddler on her lap and lean over her as though she were a tiny baby, allowing her hair to enclose the two of them and excluding the rest of the world. They would touch each other's jewelry or clothing in apparent enchantment and would recite a small repertoire of amorous play. Many treatment providers noticed that Helen would light up when discussing Dorian even at times when she demonstrated no response and registered no emotion in relation to any other subject. Helen herself stated a number of times that thoughts of Dorian were the only things that made her hesitate to die, and a number of nurses and counselors requested that Dorian's father bring her for frequent visits because she appeared to represent the single thread connecting Helen to life.

When she did not interact with Dorian in this enraptured manner, however, Helen appeared barely to be aware of the child's existence. She once went onto the patio of a psychiatric ward to smoke a cigarette in spite of the fact that Dorian did not want her mother to leave her during their visit. Dorian, who rarely demonstrated distress in such direct ways, cried inconsolably while Helen sat outside watching her through a glass wall. Helen later described this scene as "cute." Another time Dorian told everyone in the elevator and hallways on the way to the ward that she was going to "visit Mama." When she arrived she found Helen bandaged heavily because of a recent cutting episode and too depressed to lift her head from her pillow to acknowledge Dorian. Dorian retreated into

a corner facing the wall and when the therapist addressed her, responded with a whispered "Baby alone."

Helen was at times able to articulate the fact that her depressive sense of her own badness was inextricably bound up with her
belief that she was a "bad mother," and that at such moments
visits with or thoughts of Dorian exacerbated her inward collapse.
When Dorian was 3½, Helen had exhausted the county's mental
health resources and was admitted to the state psychiatric hospital for long-term treatment.

Gary and Dorian

Gary cared for Dorian increasingly during her first year of life and
exclusively as Helen spent more and more time in treatment. Gary
was 28 years old at the time of Dorian's birth. His own childhood
had been characterized by poverty and parental alcoholism, physical abuse, abandonment, and a few stints in foster care. He described
without affect periods of as long as a week during which he and his
siblings, all latency-aged, were left to fend for themselves when his
mother and stepfather, without explanation, did not appear at home.
He also remembered riding buses around town during the day rather
than attending school.

Although he had some skill in a number of trades, he worked
sporadically throughout his life and was supported by government
child support payments after Dorian's birth. He rose to the occasion of navigating (although never predicting) the incessant crises
of Helen's suicide attempts as well as his own evictions and turbulent relations with members of his extended family. His days were
organized entirely around the visiting schedules of Helen's various
treatment settings. Even under circumstances of extreme duress,
such as a rehospitalization following a hopeful period of apparent
improvement, he went to great lengths to keep the peace and to
accommodate Helen's requests for visits. Anger and upset on his
part appeared only as redoubled efforts toward accommodating

others or, at times, passive withdrawal in the form of forgetting plans, getting lost, or being too broke to travel.

With Dorian, Gary was tender in a fraternal way but oblivious when it came to understanding or responding to her internal states. This difficulty was exacerbated by the fact that he took pride in what he described as her "independence," including her indiscriminate sociability ("she's not shy or afraid of people"). Gary was similarly proud of the fact that at the age of 2 Dorian would walk five miles through the city to visit her mother at the hospital, making the trek without being carried and without complaint. Her father reported that Dorian did not cry when she got bumped or scratched in a fall the way other children did. Although he had been worried for her safety, he delighted in telling the story of Dorian at the age of 3 walking away from him in a movie theater. He had finally found her seated in the front row of the dark theater completely engrossed in the movie. Within the treatment, Gary sought the therapist's approval for his parenting of Dorian, anxiously reporting details of her diet and activities while ignoring Dorian's immediate overtures toward him for interaction.

Dorian

Dorian was a highly self-sufficient child, bright, verbal, energetic, and engaging. She learned and used adults' names quickly and initiated social contact wherever she was, although there were few reports of her interacting with other children. She was able to occupy herself in solitary play for hours, making use of whatever might be on hand to amuse herself. She was robust and athletic but invested in the trappings of femininity such as dresses, jewelry, and hair accessories as well as coy modes of interacting. She was friendly and helpful and assisted her father with cooking and laundry at age 3. She had strong ideas but would abandon them if she met with disagreement. She was ceaselessly attentive to adults without the appearance of worry that can accompany vigilance in children her age. Finally, she was composed in crises. She would ignore fresh cuts and bandages on her mother's arms, and was not visibly frightened on a psychiatric ward when a patient in restraints attempted to grab her. Once, she put her coat back on when she arrived at a half-way house to visit her mother only to find that Helen had been rehospitalized.

Psychotherapy with the Family

Signs of the costs to Dorian of her hypercompetence and self-sufficiency were immediately apparent in her self-management in treatment. There were disconcerting qualities to her style of play. She was at the same time hurried, frenzied even, and deeply engrossed in toys and activities. There was an impenetrable quality to her absorption in play fragments, and yet any pursuit could be halted or abandoned in an instant as a result of either an internal or an external stimulus, only to be immediately replaced by another urgently undertaken endeavor.

Although she was extremely attractive, talkative, and engaging, her interactive repertoire was fixed and limited rather than spontaneous and evolving. She carefully monitored adults both to avoid disappointment and to capitalize on those windows of opportunity for engagement that might become available. But even when she was able to interact with adults, her activity was highly circumscribed. She could command: "Draw a doggie here, Papa"; she could perform: "Dorian, show Maria how you do the patty-cake song"; and she could surround the therapist in play that was superficially elaborate but required little real emotional interchange: "We're eating breakfast. You want pancakes? Here's yours. You take this red plate. No, this yellow one. Here's your juice and here's my juice. We are in the jungle now! Oh-oh. There's a bear. Now go to sleep. Hey, where did that toy truck go?"

Even when her play concerned apparently highly charged themes (hospital, separations and reunions, hunger), she seemed to perform it rather than play it. She would give and request pretend shots or bandages with untiring cheerfulness. She would enact endlessly and cheerfully things being taken away just when it appeared they would be given. She would spin stories in stylized rapture (reminiscent of her enchantment games with Helen) about, for example, Snow White and the prince being cast out of castle after castle. But inquiry or interpretation on any of these subjects would call forth a brief signal of anxiety that might evoke the therapist's reaction but not lead anywhere. Instead, Dorian would hurry on to a new play fragment or just turn up the charm.

Despite these difficulties, Dorian was able to begin to trust and depend on the therapist over a number of months. As time passed, Dorian's inner struggles began to break through both within and beyond the sessions. First, in her haste and urgency during sessions, Dorian would bump into things and fall frequently. Initially she did not respond at all to these mishaps and indeed seemed startled by any adult response to them. But eventually she became confused and frightened when she hurt herself. Then she might cry but she would vehemently refuse adult help, screaming "leave me alone" if she was approached. She developed sleep disturbances, resisting falling asleep and waking up frightened. And although she had become nearly toilet trained at the age of 2, she began to lose bowel and bladder control, with periods of intermittent enuresis and encopresis. Overall, her bodily states began to show the distress that she could not otherwise articulate.

Around nine months into the treatment, she also began to have episodes of severe emotional distress with inconsolable crying and physically retreating into corners or burrowing into pieces of furniture. She was unable to be soothed in these states, again demanding in apparent rage and terror, "leave me alone." These episodes were triggered by the threat of separation (they became routine around the close of each session), or by a frustration, disappointment, or failure, such as a change in plans, a fall, or an incident of enuresis. They would be resolved by Dorian's eventually pulling herself together and passing into a state of apparent numbness, at which point she would be cooperative and compliant.

Helen was rehospitalized at one point during this phase of the treatment after a few weeks of relative consistency and calm in the external circumstances of Dorian's caregiving surround. As a result

of a misunderstanding between the therapist and Gary, it fell on
the therapist to inform Dorian of her mother's rehospitalization,
such that she would not be visiting Helen at the usual half-way house.
Dorian immediately responded by verbally contradicting the therapist ("Mama is at Jackson House") and simultaneously losing bowel
control. She proceeded through the duration of the session in a mode
of rigid friendliness, at once denying that she had soiled herself and
complying with her father's efforts in cleaning and changing her.

The next week, Gary phoned the therapist to say that he would
be unable to bring Dorian to her session. Dorian asked to speak
with the therapist and said on the telephone, "I want to come to
where you work." Gary did bring Dorian the next week and the
session unfolded as follows:

> Dorian stands at the office door, hesitating to come in. She scowls
> at the therapist through the door. Gary hurries her in. The thera-
> pist comments that it looks like Dorian didn't want to hurry in today.
> Dorian is already busy cooking for the therapist, ignoring her father.
> The therapist and Gary review the arrangement for the session and
> Gary departs, as is customary during this phase of the treatment.
> Dorian refuses to say good-bye to Gary.
>
> She is already playing in a hyper-energized way. She announces
> that it is the therapist's birthday and she sings happy birthday to her.
> She also gives the therapist a present of some playroom dishes inside
> a cloth bag. She feeds the therapist pretend pancakes and says, "Here's
> your pancakes!" The therapist replies, "Thank you. These are yummy!"
> Dorian says, "Here's your juice in the blue cup . . . No, you get the red
> cup. I get the blue cup." The therapist says, "Thank you for the juice.
> You're making us quite a breakfast." Dorian asks whether the thera-
> pist likes pancakes, and she answers, "I like pancakes a lot!"
>
> Dorian then puts her cheek on the arm of the therapist's chair
> and says, "I love you Maria." The therapist responds, "You want me
> to know about your love. And also I think I'm getting all these pres-
> ents and food and love because you are worried that I'm mad at
> you." Dorian corrects her, "No *I* am mad at *you*." The therapist says,
> "Ah-ha. We had such a hard good-bye last time and then we didn't
> see each other for a long long time." Dorian prompts, "Open your
> present, Maria." Therapist: "What's inside?" Dorian: "Mad at you."

The therapist pulls out a plate and asks, "Is this mad-at-you?" Dorian: "Yes!" Dorian puts the plate halfway across the floor. The therapist observes, "I see you're putting mad-at-you very far away." Dorian explains, "So it doesn't bother you." Therapist: "You are worried that mad-at-you will bother me."

Dorian goes to the table to get crayons. "This one is mad," she announces. "This one is mad too. This one is happy. NO! It's mad." She becomes distressed—she has dropped all the crayons off the table onto the floor. The therapist says, "So many crayons. It's hard to find a crayon that isn't mad today." Dorian amplifies the idea, "Mad crayons!" She moves to stomp on them. The therapist says, "I'm not going to let you break the crayons but I see that you want them way down under the table and you want to crush them." Dorian: "Bad crayons. Bad mad crayons. Dead." She pushes them farther under the table. The therapist says, "You think the mad crayons are bad. They are far, far away and dead."

Dorian switches abruptly, saying, "You Jasmine I Snow White. Jasmine, call your mom." Therapist complies, "Rrring. Hello? Mom?" Dorian: "Yes, Baby." Therapist: "What should I say?" Dorian; "Say 'I love you Mom.'" Therapist: "I love you Mom." Dorian: "I love you Baby." Therapist asks, "What should I say now?" Dorian repeats the same script and this caricatured conversation is repeated several times. Then Dorian announces, "I'm calling my mom. Hello, Mom. OK." She is speaking now in a busy, impenetrable mode. "I'm the mom. I'm mad." Therapist: "The mom is mad?" Dorian: "No, happy. You the daddy. You mad." Therapist: "Kind of confusing—so many people who are maybe mad." Dorian: "No, I'm the teacher. I'm making pancakes. You want pancakes?" Therapist (winded): "Sure."

A familiar cooking and feeding episode ensues. Dorian wants the therapist here exactly. No, here. No, in this chair. Dorian moves her own chair right over the spot where she lost bowel control last week. She barricades herself and the therapist into this corner with chairs. She stuffs all the cooking supplies onto the shelves. The therapist asks, "Aren't those shelves getting pretty full?" Dorian insists "No." A pot falls from a shelf. Dorian anxiously puts it back. Therapist: "You are very worried that I will be mad if there's a mess?" Dorian: "There is no mess. You want more pancakes?"

The therapist reminds Dorian, "Soon we will hear the doorbell and then your papa will come in." Dorian gets the baby doll and commands, "Cover her up. She mad at you. She don't want to look at you." The therapist says, "She is so mad at me she doesn't want to look at me." Dorian: "No, she happy at you." Therapist: "I know sometimes babies are mad at me and happy at me all at the same time. That's very confusing for babies."

Now Dorian commands, "Take off her dress." The therapist complies, narrating "You want her dress off." Dorian: "Take off her pants. She's gonna be naked. Take off her socks." The therapist undresses the doll and observes, "The baby is naked." Dorian takes the doll from the therapist and reports, "She pooped on her pants. The daddy is mad. Bad baby, you pooped on your socks." Therapist: "The baby pooped and the daddy is mad?" Dorian: "Bad baby." Therapist: "The baby must be scared and sad and mad and embarrassed." Dorian: "Bad baby."

Therapist: "You think the baby is very bad. Maybe you think it was very bad when you pooped the last time and maybe you worry that I was mad at you." Dorian: "No, *you* pooped and I was mad at *you*." Therapist: "It was very confusing with all that poop and all those mad feelings."

Gary arrives and Dorian becomes distressed around the leave-taking. She doesn't want to relinquish certain toys or put her coat on. She retreats to a corner and says, "Leave me alone." The therapist says, "This is a hard time for you. Do you know that we will say goodbye differently today? Usually you and your papa go through the door and I stay here in the playroom. Today I will go through the door with you and your papa and we will go see your mama. Then I will say good-bye to you there." This organizes and calms her. She makes sure, "You and me and Papa go through the door and go see Mama?" The therapist says "Yes." The three depart together.

DISCUSSION

At first glance and at some distance, Dorian's social dexterity and her apparently articulate play may seem to reflect her obvious intelligence and canny resilience. She shows, as in this hour, a capacity to talk about and play with difficult themes that seem to represent some of the agonizing issues of a little girl in her situation.

She is apparently poised, charming and sociable, agile with words and symbols, and able to handle all sorts of challenges. But her competencies are organized in a stoic and rigid way that keeps others at a distance and avoids the possibility of softness and dependency. With detached deftness, she uses her verbal abilities and social skills to sustain a brittle and often driven and manic-like aura.

In the session, she uses her substantial abilities to verbalize, play, and construct story fragments in a series of valiant but tenuous efforts to contain profound desires and anxieties that beleaguer her. Angry and persecuted feelings break through all over; poignant longings to be comforted, to be fed and to love and be loved flow through the session in various, often inchoate forms; and the mortification associated with the previous session's loss of bowel control lurks just beyond the horizon. Beneath the apparently composed surface of her precocious style, an array of anxieties threatens to break through and overwhelm her. She is profoundly uneasy about separation, attachment, aggression, and persecution. But rather than experiencing these issues as distinct wishes with associated dangers, she is uncertain and unformed at her core. In a brittle and alienated effort to manage the approach of very difficult emotional and interpersonal realities, Dorian's intelligence and facility with toys and words serve to keep her at a distance from the authentic, but overwhelming dimensions of her inner life. She cannot find a secure resting place.

Neither of Dorian's parents has provided a matrix in which her infantile feelings, vulnerabilities, and perceptions can be recognized, appreciated, and integrated into meaning and responsiveness. Instead, it is capacities, not affects or authentic play, that one finds when meeting Dorian; she is always challenged to cope, to be sociable, deft, and cute and to do whatever is necessary. But no space has been left for her to be an infant. Activity is highly energized for Dorian, but this very energy becomes a shield against the external world and her inner turbulence rather than a way to engage and transform them. Her apparent enthusiasm protects her from real engagement with her inner world and external actualities, and she struggles to maintain omnipotence and detachment.

In her traumatic world, Dorian has few opportunities to develop an authentic sense of herself. She is poignantly concerned with her mother, subjected to the most radical and trying swings of her mother's availability, depression, and aggression, and has been offered little help to make sense of this turbulent and primitive attachment. Subjected to extraordinary inconsistency by Helen, Dorian has been at the mercy of her mother's malignant and depressive projections at the same time as she has been called upon to become suffused in idealizations that have had little to do with how it feels to be a baby. Helen uses Dorian to fill her own longings and crumbling sense of self. In a sense, Dorian has been responsible for her mother's life. Alternatively, Helen's self-hating idea that she is a bad and hateful person and mother submerges Dorian.

Both the good and bad projections arise and are imposed on Dorian, without regard to her own inner states, needs, affects, and anxieties. In such an atmosphere, in order to have a relationship with her mother at all, Dorian is overwhelmed, never feeling a sense of her own integrity and agency, and being pressed to find a way to accommodate these various projections, to accompany her mother in them, and to handle, somehow, the shattering external unpredictabilities and internal fears and inconsistencies that they must induce in her. The wild and dramatic episodes observed in the inpatient unit, ranging from Helen's engulfing Dorian in her hair to cruelly ignoring her screams while smoking her cigarette, would be unbearable for even the most psychologically competent adult. Indeed, most of the therapists who have been subjected to Helen's torturous and "manipulative" behaviors have given up. But these patterns have been at the core of Dorian's earliest experiences, and she has had no choice, no other world.

When Helen leaves so little room for Dorian's own experience, identification with projections fills the space more optimally occupied by transformational, creative, vitalizing response and recognition. It is hard to imagine what a true self would mean for Dorian, since in her core relationship with her mother she has always had to exercise the most vigilant attention to the other's state of mind in order to stay in whatever kind of contact is possible. One can imagine an absorptive "taking on" of the mother's states—a primitive kind of what is sometimes crudely called incorporation, but is more accurately rendered in terms of a kind of pressured, responsive immersion in the mother's experience at the expense of her own.

For an infant, this could take the form of a special and careful attention to her mother's moods, postures, physical expressions, and the like—a precursor of Dorian's social hyperattentiveness. Similarly, special efforts to communicate and to grasp and energize the communicative process might also follow, along with an attempt to pay special attention and invest extra energy in those internal representations that hold the memory of such satisfying interactions as had taken place. But such efforts would only lead to fleeting security, a rhythm of special efforts to sustain what is good that can only be briefly kept up and will crumble when challenged, either by other internal information or external impingements, like the therapist's attempts at empathic interpretation in the above hour.

Dorian's relationship with her father offered no substantial alternative to this insecurity and disorganization. In their everyday routines, he has praised her for meeting demands usually assigned to those years older than she, such as walking miles across the city or spending days camping in the wilderness, and she has learned endurance and stoicism as a core element of what it means to be with someone else. The shallowness of her father's appreciation of her resourcefulness does not provide enough to reassure her, especially mixed as it is with his own ambivalence, depression, and pervasive and passive ineffectuality. Although Dorian's father has been more stable than her mother and cares for her in a much more reliable and straightforward way, he cannot see her agonies—only her capacities. He has offered her no authentic experience of love, recognition, or mutual influence. He has been dedicated to the pragmatic side of her connection with Helen, but is unable to offer any help with the emotional. For him, this is more or less the way the world works, and despite how much he cares for his daughter, he sees no reason why it should be different for her.

Gary has thus left Dorian emotionally stranded with her tormented and tormenting mother. But at the same time, their relationship has further influenced her particular styles of handling and turning away from her anxieties by celebrating her self-sufficiency. This encouragement also supports her identifying with his way of just getting along. This identification is the straightforward type of adopting the attributes of the one to whom one is attached, as opposed to the mix of accepting projections and hypervigilant absorption that blends with imitation in Dorian's relationship with Helen.

One is left with the impression of a little girl working hard to find an equilibrium who can never actually relax enough to let her guard down. It is the activity itself—the exercise of capacities—that becomes the guardian of whatever safety and relatedness can be secured. In a kind of proto-intellectualization, symbolic and social activity are energized in themselves and become an arena where a vulnerable mode of safety is briefly and transiently secured. In embracing activity, Dorian is tenuously asserting her own pseudo-autonomy and imperviousness, providing as it does the best alternative to having nothing at all, or perhaps worse, the crazy torturousness of her mother. At the same time, her omnipotence and constant doing reproduce her mother's more histrionic, demanding, and oppressive way of controlling her objects. For Dorian, it is as if activity and competence can take the place of reality; the adaptive capacity itself becomes the object, rather than mediating between the subject and her objects. Relational space is thus collapsed, and the ego is energized in a deadened, rather than vitalizing manner.

The driven expediency of this style becomes more obvious when the poignant wishes that lie behind it emerge for a moment ("I want to go where you work") or even more dramatically, in moments of breakdown such as crying, falling, or enuresis and encopresis. This is most dramatically illustrated when Dorian loses control of her bowels at the clinic after she learns that she will not see her mother. She tries to insist that her mother will be available, but despite her formidable verbal dexterity, she cannot succeed in making reality other than what it is. Instead, her body insists on the truth, and she explodes in the face of her profound anxieties about her mother's disappearance. This is a terribly poignant breakdown of her usu-

ally successful, if brittle, efforts to use words and her other precocious coping abilities to omnipotently create her own pseudo-reality
rather than to link herself to the one that is out there and shared
by others. Her usually successful imperviousness is shattered when
the harsher realities of her interpersonal world remind her of their
indifference to her needs and wishes. Her frequent falls may be
similarly construed, where her constant effort at keeping the world
at a distance ends in a moment where her sense of being off balance literally comes through.

The Hour

In this hour, Dorian's activity has a frenetic, hyperenergized and
brittle quality that may give the casual observer the impression that
she is involved with the "important" themes, but mostly embodies
her omnipotent, single-minded effort to keep things moving and keep
the therapist at a distance. The therapist's persistent efforts to think
with Dorian are repeatedly deflected. Sometimes they are pushed
aside and at other times they are transformed destructively or incorporated without being heard. By deft use of verbalization, play,
and the tactics of narrative construction she *plays out* her sense of
being desperately off-balance and hungry, but she cannot stop to
feel what it is like to be these ways. Dorian skirts her fears and
desires, rather than experiencing them.

Prior to the hour and at a distance, Dorian has been able to make
a real declaration of her love for Maria, but in her presence, she is
reluctant and scowling. She then shifts to try to make reparation,
with an exaggerated and precocious tone, cooking like a grownup,
inventing a birthday, and coquettishly declaring her love.

Here, as throughout the session, Dorian is adopting the role
usually taken by the adult—feeding the therapist and giving her a
present, and one sees how she works to obscure her own needs by
becoming the one to whom she would look for satisfaction of them.
Much in Dorian's play here seems to correspond to the absorbent

hyperattentiveness to her mother described earlier. It is also a way of acting as if she were older than she is, and has the "as-if" quality typical of much of Dorian's sociability and play.

Dorian here is identifying with both wished-for and feared others. She cannot tolerate the differentiation normally expected of children her age, since it would expose her to basic and very troubling feelings of rejection and deprivation. Instead, she takes the place of the object rather than modifying an already established self-representation, and thus blurs the distinction between herself and her objects. In doing this, she eludes her own inner world and acts out a role. This style of identifying is quite different from those that embody the absence or loss of the other; this one cancels out the difference between the subjectivity of the person and the otherness of her objects, rather than being organized around an internal representation of a two-person relationship, where a distinct self-representation is modified to become more like another.

Dorian's use of identifications in this hour, then, offers some unusual insight into the ways in which an infant forms an identity in her relationships with her parents. These processes are more complex than what is usually captured in the emphasis on identification as a process by which the individual's self-image is modified to become more like the other person (Sandler and Rosenblatt 1962). Most treatments of the subject of identification take the structure of the self-object distinction as already given, prior to the identificatory transformation of the self-representation. In Dorian, however, identification is a mode in which the basic structures of self and other are themselves being formed and delineated, and their relation to one another is organized as she takes on and molds to her mother's demands. On a conceptual level, such identifications must be understood not just as modifications of a preexisting "self," but as processes in which the contours, boundaries, and mental locations of the experiences of self and object become organized at the most basic level of psychic structure.

Along such lines, Dorian's way of putting herself in the place of the other suggests something of how she handles and structures boundaries between herself and others. Dislocation, anxiety, and indefiniteness underlie the superficial sense that she is able to manage the space between herself and others. In the face of her mother's projective and overwhelming onslaughts on her inner world, and lacking recognition or a space for her own unrepresented affects, needs, and bodily experiences to take on any meaning, she is left to make exaggerated efforts to create herself in the place of the other. This effort, even at its most successful, leaves her in an uncertain and only vaguely organized state of insecurity and pseudo-relatedness, such that the moving into the other's place, whether aggressor or caregiver, has a secondary purpose. In a kind of exaggerated identification, Dorian does away with her worrying wishes and fears, especially her longings for love and her fears of being attacked and abandoned. Here, identification serves defensive purposes while having the more global effect of forming an inauthentic, self-alienated experience.

Another identification maneuver follows the therapist's speculation that Dorian is afraid that she, Maria, is angry at her. Dorian again identifies with the object, this time the persecutory introjected aggressor, and says "No, *I* am mad at *you!*" But this frightening affect is, finally, not contained, and Dorian regressively and distressingly erupts, using the crayons in a concrete way that suggests the more primitive contours of her inner world that underlie the precocious container that has now thinned out. She works desperately to get rid of the bad things, and the explosion is reminiscent of the previous bowel movement.

Maria now makes an effort to get Dorian to stop destroying the crayons. Whereas on some other occasions this therapist might have been more likely to allow a young child to proceed with her regression and aggression, Maria here has a sense of the intensity of Dorian's primitive destructiveness, as well as the torments that her mother has shared with her. In an ambitious effort that is both supportive and interpretive, Maria hopes that Dorian will feel protected and reassured by being restrained; at the same time, she hopes that Dorian will be able to make use of an effort to put her angry feeling into words.

But this does not rescue her, and Dorian remains disorganized with her primitive, basic, almost structureless aggressivity continuing on the surface. She finally extricates herself, as she has in the past, by an abrupt change in the subject ("You Jasmine. I Snow White.") Jasmine now calls her mom; Dorian is her mom, and gets to live out the longed-for love of her mother, maintaining herself in an omnipotent and impenetrable stance toward the therapist. Perhaps she is recalling the early moments of submersion in her mother's idealizations.

But this is a short-lived respite. Again, the anger breaks through, and Dorian has to scramble to keep herself whole. Again, she plays the role of the adult, feeding Maria. Dorian does what she can to experience a feeding, even if she cannot bear to be the hungry one. As in the beginning of the hour, she regressively evokes themes associated with an earlier developmental stage, but she must exert firm control over Maria and then extend the same effort to cramming the pots and pans in the shelves. Noticing that this is the same spot as the "pooping" episode and guessing that Dorian is trying to undo the previous outburst, the therapist talks about a mess. Dorian fends this off and again offers food, but she soon returns to the theme, undressing the doll-baby who has pooped on her pants and socks.

There are glimmers of authenticity and inwardness to this passage, along with a direct, if delayed, response to the previous interpretation. Still, Dorian promptly takes the role of the critic, and makes Maria the one who pooped. Dorian's facility at playing serves her typical effort to fend off or alter reality to protect her tenuous inner world.

A Note on Technique

As Gary arrives and the hour ends, Dorian's reluctance to leave Maria becomes more apparent. But she is reassured to learn that they will all go see her mother. That Dorian is so responsive to direct reassurance raises a question about the therapist's technique in this hour, which has some implications for technique in such cases in general. Many of the interventions are efforts to direct Dorian's attention to the anxious feelings and self-images, notably her being "mad," out of control of a mess, and seen as bad for making the mess. These are fairly deep and somewhat intellectual interpretations, not so typical of therapies of traumatized children. They often make Dorian anxious and lead to abrupt shifts in focus and a general defensiveness. At times, these comments do appear to lead her to move closer to the theme that is offered, within a few moments if not immediately.

Since Dorian often does not consistently appear to make direct use of these interventions, we are led to ask, in retrospect, whether alternative approaches might have been more effective. Perhaps direct reassurance would have been useful in relieving her anxiety, as it seemed to be at the end of the meeting. Would it have been more helpful to go along even more with Dorian's efforts to play out situations where she felt safe, by, for example, helping Dorian get rid of the "bad, mad" crayons in a safe place? Along similar lines, the therapist might have embraced roles offered by Dorian, such as taking the role of the baby when Dorian calls her in the middle of the session. This might involve, for example, saying, "Oh, Mom, I'm so happy you called." Some effort to deepen the emotional contact might now be offered in such contexts (as by adding, in this example, "I missed you and I was worried about you . . ."). A third approach might have involved more commenting on Dorian's anxieties, saying something about, for instance, how hard some of these things must be to think about. Instead, the therapist has a tendency to step outside of the play and make some effort to talk with Dorian from the position of an observer and to probe through the resistances rather than flowing with them.

Finding the best approach is difficult under the easiest of circumstances, and especially so with younger children, when the environment is so unsupportive and when the anxieties are as treacherous as they are for Dorian. Although at times this approach is successful in this hour, there may be something gained from examining, in retrospect and such as we can, what led to the relatively interpretive approach here.

Certain special conditions occur in cases such as Dorian's that make such precocious technique more likely. Dorian's play, for instance, seems so articulate and she seems so willing to talk about the things that are bothering her that it seems natural to intervene at the more verbal and deep levels. In addition, she would rarely allow the therapist to soothe her, and would generally be unavailable, or only intermittently available, to the more ordinary approaches. This prods her therapist to make the special effort involved in pushing through to some of her deeper concerns.

The extra investment in a communicating mode that is somewhat detached and verbally dexterous parallels, in a rough way, Dorian's precocious position in standing outside of her own emotional life and at some detachment from the immediacy of the personal, interpersonal, and even physical realities that characterize her developmental environment. It seems reasonable to think that the therapist's style is in some way complementary to and responsive to Dorian's. Some have indeed remarked that "precocious patients pull for precocious technique" (see Corrigan and Gordon, Chapter 1, this volume). In other words, Dorian's overreliance on symbolic processes stimulates a similar reaction in her therapist and perhaps in others around her. This is how Dorian gives herself shape, and an even more special effort would be required to find a way to fit with her that does not conform to her alienated and defensive presentation.

REFERENCES

Fraiberg, S., ed. (1980). *Clinical Studies in Infant Mental Health: The First Year of Life.* New York: Basic Books.

Lieberman, A. F., and Pawl, J. H. (1993). Infant–parent psychotherapy. In *Handbook of Infant Mental Health*, ed. C. H. Zeanah. New York: Guilford.

Sandler, J., and Rosenblatt, B. (1962). The concept of the representational world. *Psychoanalytic Study of the Child* 17:128–145. New York: International Universities Press.

Seligman, S. (1994). Applying psychoanalysis in an unconventional context. Adapting infant–parent psychotherapy to a changing population. *Psychoanalytic Study of the Child* 49:481–500. New Haven, CT: Yale University Press.

9

Of Two Minds: The Mind's Relation with Itself

Harold N. Boris

Ultimately was a location Harpur always tried to skirt.
—Bill James, *Protection*

It was one of those periods of the analysis, about five years in, during which I was feeling I had for the while said everything and could only unnecessarily repeat myself. My patient, although as always informative and cooperative, was, I sensed, feeling fearful and envious, anyway reluctant, but I didn't know what else to say. Occasionally wisps of something to say would drift through my thoughts, but none of these seemed contributive, and I didn't want to work at formulating them. I must have said so, something like, "I think there is something possibly to be said, but I can't yet see what it might be." It was then that he took a certain pity on me.

With great diffidence, ready to stop on the instant lest he was trespassing or worse, telling me something I already knew, he noted for me that although the paintings on the walls of my consulting room were, in the manner of Braque or Matisse, flat still lifes, I had recently put vases quite like those that were in the paintings themselves on each of the tables that stood in front of the paintings. In the newly added vases were arrays of silk or dried flowers, just as there were flowers in the vases in the pictures. The effects, he averred, were twofold: to take what was flat and (as it were) two-dimensional and make it three-dimensional, and to point up the flatness of the objects in the painting. Here he paused for me to see the points.

When he felt I had had time to do so, he assured me he didn't feel the implication of this change in furnishing had been contrived exclusively for him or even wholly intended as a communication. But although the medium of the message was subtle, the message itself was not: I was getting sick and tired of his two-position universe.

The expression *two-position universe* was one I had coined for referring to my patient's propensity to take any and every event as one in which one person was doing something to another. It had elements of the paranoid/schizoid position in which splittings and projections are prominent. There were never more than two players at a time, and if one wasn't doing something to the other, the other was doing something to the first. At heart it expressed his wish to undiscover the mother in order to have unimpeded access to the breast. This was not in itself so triangular as it might seem; the breast to which he wanted unalloyed access was his own, untrammeled by the sort of self-conscious that Winnicott (1971) described: "The mother is looking at the baby and what she looks like is what she sees there" (p. 112), which is to say what he looks like is what he sees there. I used the expression to display insofar as I could that in so constructing the world, he opened himself to great fear, exaggerated ideas of impact, and great envy. I also used it to try to display how that configuration evaded anything like a three-person world with its oedipal triumphs and disappointments. Sometimes he could make use of this characterization, revisit what he had been (almost) experiencing and find the three-person world that had gotten obscured and abandoned. Sometimes all he could relate to was what he felt he had done to me or what I was doing to him.

From one eye, I could see that his description of the meaning inhering in my placement of the round jugs with their jolly flowers was his evocation, even his reassertion of the two-position universe. From the other I could see that he worried lest there might have been changes in me that, if I didn't know about, hence couldn't reconsider, I would be unable to protect him from. He counted on my willingness to take care of my emotions toward him. I said something like, "You must have been afraid for your mind—that I have taken to working on it," and he nodded.

I was interested that, rather than speaking, he nodded, and that, rather than looking at the vases and paintings or into the woods, through the great bay window I had recently installed, I looked at him in time to catch the nod. I had made him see. He had required me to see. Seeing in conjunction with the jugs suggested an interpretation about breasts, but such an interpretation at that moment would have seemed a further attack on his mind. What need had he for a mind of such subtlety only to have it felled by the Breast? The disguise was transparent, but so are all the *haute* creations of Paris and Milan. Would one say to Lagerfeld, "So what do we have here, a dress of some sort?" The breast, moreover, was a source without favor. All the same I felt annoyed by what for the moment I felt as his preciosity.

The *subject*, or naive and un-self-reflexive, mind comes about, so I think, as a result of natural selection: out of a reservoir of protomental potentia, the environment invites and requires some, not all, of what is in the pool.[1] We do not respond to the environment by learning—by inventing and contriving adaptive responses to the stimulus. Rather the responses are there, latent until called upon. The environment does not teach us how to respond; it educates us in the original sense of leading or bringing out. Gerald Edelman (1987) has compared this to the way the infective agent selects the particulars of the possible immunological response. Damasio (1994)

---

1. Natural selection has been understood and misunderstood to consist only of the chance effects of the agencies of predation, drought, and the landfall of asteroids upon the fate of the then extant creatures. Understood, because there is a contingent element in the weeding and pruning of creatures within species as well as entire species themselves. (Perhaps 0.06 percent of all species survive today.) Misunderstood, because selection also takes place within a species via the systematic choosing of whom shall mate when and with whom; and by which offspring shall survive and which be subject to predation or neglect. (This is sometimes quite intricate: later hatched chicks have a greater amount of chemical energizers in their eggs so that though younger and smaller at hatching they can compete with the others already in the clutch.) But it is not often or comfortably thought that the mind is formed and shaped by the same "Darwinian" system.

writes, "Dispositional representations exist in a potential state, subject to activation . . . like the town of Brigadoon." The quiet, unfettered unfoldings of mind are to many an experience of vast delight: the reverie, the brown study, the ideational slipstream, the gentle ticking over of mentation. Ogden's (1994) word for this is *rumination* and he compares this to an autistic shape:

> Relations with autistic shapes and objects are "perfect" in that they lie outside of the unpredictability of relations with human beings. . . . These "felt shapes" and "felt objects" exist outside of time and place. I would like to focus for illustrative purposes on rumination as a use of ideation as an autistic shape. Rumination is a form of mental activity that can be called upon instantaneously as a sensory medium in which one can immerse oneself. [It] serves to protect the individual against the continuous strain that is an inescapable part of living in the unpredictable matrix of human object relations. . . . Rumination can be compared to a flawlessly operating machine. Nothing in the world of object relations can be compared to it. [pp. 175–176]

And yet, and yet. The problem for the *object* mind—that self-reflexive mind we take as our other, our object—is that this subject mind is being created, selected, edited, pasted, and published—without it having much say in the matter. It remembers things we might prefer to forget and forgets what we would like to remember. So too does it see, hear, smell, and taste, does it long for, desire, loathe, and fear not that to which we have chosen to attend but that which nevertheless has chosen us. The environment that selects us is everywhere—from our brain and its neuronal firings to our body with its busy chemical messaging, to everything that impinges from outside our skins, both proximate and at long range. Our minds are formed before we have a cortex with which to think. The universe, that is, is an *influencing machine* (Tausk 1919): Unless we are careful, we will be as "educated" as Lorenz's (1965) goslings were imprinted by his Wellington boots. Vases appear in front of paintings. Influences abound.

To the mind, the source of the influence is often perplexing; whence comes the particular selections? Since the infant directs his or her own attempts at influencing the mother—selecting, or trying to, from among her repertoire of responses—it is likely to seem as if the influences flow from her. And so, to a great extent, they do. (But as we know from people closely in touch with their psychotic natures, influence also flows from "it" or "them.") The response from the infant is to try the harder to influence the source of the influence, to establish and convey at least an exchange. If he or she cannot, the other is experienced as persecutory, this no matter the nature of the influences, which in and of themselves might be benign. Any influence that is not allowed by the other to be reciprocal excites hatred and envy and inspires an attack on the link.[2]

Additional perplexity arises as to the nature of the persecution: Is it the influencing—the appearance of the vases? Or is it the lack of reciprocal receptivity—my closed-mindedness to the importance to my patient of his two-position universe? The object mind now comes about to invigilate this worrisome process. It stands in for both the mind of the other and for the subject mind. It becomes, in this, a variant of the transitional object. It is designed to be temporary, but it may have to endure, blocking the growth of mutual and collaborative thought. Coltart's patient does not seem—at first—so much to miss her during separations as to hate her power to impose them; he responds with sadomasochistic envy. Later, as he comes into connections with his hates and loves, and his insomnia eases, he yearns for union and reunion. Still later, he appears to be with her in fantasy: his contribution to the charity with which she was affiliated seems to say, Remember me? I have not forgotten you. Oh, how I have not forgotten you.

My patient could not really understand what we were doing together if we were not trying to effect selection. Why else would we be together? What else were we trying to do?

If, as I prefer, we think of mind as an integral of possibles—possible ideas, possible feelings, possible intentions—some of which the

---

2. We know that analyses falter or even founder in proportion to the analyst's unwillingness to become subject to the influences of the patient without fear or so much hatred as to cause the analyst to retaliate.

forces of its environs animate and vivify, such forces show up as a
thump on the carapace of the system. They set the mind to reeling,
after which it settles, as it were, into a new configuration. It is of no
little conceptual importance to differentiate this from learning or
mapping. There is no one-to-one correlation between what one is
taught and what one "learns." Between the stimulus and the response lies the integral system of one's mental world. When that
world seems important, one goes ahead and creates a mind to super-
intend the subject mind. This is the *object* mind.

The object mind arises in order to see to it that the subject mind
is not made subject to the will and whim of the contingent universe.
Here come the first small paroxysms of willful being; Spitz (1957),
following Freud (1925) on negation, said the ego was formed upon
the word *no*. As the self, having come into being upon the tides of
self-consciousness, begins its first tentative strut upon the heights,
part of what it surveys is the clickety click of mind. I think therefore, I yam. Just as there is a moment in time when our recollections include us as a person in the remembered scenes, there is a
moment when mind reflects on mind. To many this does not seem
to be an event of moment; to some, such as the various patients
who have become the subjects of this volume of essays, this first
encounter with their own mentality is momentous.

My patient was fond of telling a story on himself: One particularly fine day he went to a take-out gourmet sandwich shop and
treated himself to a Turkey Delight. A block later, chomping away,
he said to himself: "Do you realize? There is nothing but ham and
cheese in your Turkey Delight!" This little story was, of course, a
parable about his fate, his typical brand of luck. But he also used it
to evince the need for vigilance—not only or even so much against
careless shopkeepers and other providers, but of his own susceptible nature; the entire block he walked before he could discern
the ham and cheese from the Turkey Delight. The vases.

Mind as object of self comes into self's employ and provides a
degree of autonomy (or the illusion of autonomy); we now make up
our minds about this or that—or so we think and like to think. What
perforce we had to experience, we can now alter. We can establish

screens with which to obscure the original imprint; we link this with that and form analogues, and with analogies we can think syllogistically and symbolically. This newly empowered object mind sets at bay the immediate impacts of the environment. Ultimately, the mind as object is defined by such an analogy (for example, the mind questing for autonomy trying to free itself of shame and doubt may be based on an anal analogy; it arises, developmentally, at much the same time[3]). If the writer calls his book his baby, what does he call his mind? There are occasions, however, when once fashioned, an analogy destroys its logos. The originator still calls his project his brainchild, but neither of them remembers with any accuracy what a baby is (Boris 1994b). Too often people become too good at what they are good at.

Object in psychoanalysis has taken on the meaning of "other," usually another person, and when I write of the mind as object, this is the sense in which I use the word. The self, the I, the subject mind, take the object mind as its other. But I am not talking so much of self here, as of mind. When the supervening or object mind is in place, and able to some degree to introduce countervailing activity against the somewhat influence-bound disposition of the subject mind, it becomes available as an object. That is, the cleavage between the subject mind and the object mind, although it originates in the need to get beyond being educated and onto learning and imagining, forms the division that then makes an object relationship between the two minds possible. Such a relationship requires that something naively unified—mind—be sundered into two or more representations.

There is a mentality that leads us to look at the world with an eye to seeing differences, between which reciprocal libidinal relationships can be formed. In an extended work on the subject (Boris 1993) I have come to call this process COUPLING. COUPLING has as its motto *vive la différence!* Having two of anything, each different from

---

3. Harold Stewart's woman patient (Chapter 3) illustrates the struggle between doubt and belief, submission and defiance, assertion and symbiosis. Can we suspect the same of the "ancient rock" with whom (which?) Stewart nobly struggles to give empathic realization?

the other, offers possibilities for relationships that are fashioned by exchanging *different* qualities, for example, mouth–breast, man–woman; in the analytic situation, COUPLING is expressed in the transference and countertransference. The reverse trend is PAIRING. PAIRING thrives on the commonalities that facilitate identifications. Two or more naively disparate objects are considered with an eye to discovering similarities or identities, in order to be taken as if they were one. This agglomeration serves certain needs arising from the wish to relate to others by merging, fusing or mutually identifying; it comprises the identification portion of projective identifications. PAIRING is the way we express and realize our membership in groups and societies: out of many, one. You will see from this that I consider both tropes present from the inception and responsible for the ways the world is discovered and interpreted. Thus, in the COUPLE mentality, three make for an Oedipus complex, in the PAIR mentality, for a group. The same holds true of the configurations of whole and part internal objects. The breast my patient yearned for when in the two-position universe was PAIR-shaped; he wanted to put into (in the COUPLE sense) more than to take from. Instead he had to be content with the split out of which he contrived his object mind.

In its way, the formation of such an out-of-one, two relationship between the minds undoes the immense work that may have gone into the formation of any previous conception that the mind (or other organ) is a unified and cohesive part of self—that the stomach-ache, for example, isn't an object in the sense that the breast is. But when the subject mind is too suggestible, too susceptible to influences and impressions, the individual may feel this disestablishment appears to be worth it.

There is much to be investigated concerning the attributes and representations of the object mind; it can be based on hope, as within the PAIRING motive, and subserve narcissistic needs. Mimesis is an important element in this striving. It can stand in for an other in such a way as to provide the other half of an object relation based on COUPLING, as, that is, a libidinal object in which the differences that serve the wish to COUPLE are featured. Or it can be seen as an aspect, split out or split off, of the subject mind; whether it is split "out," as a specialization of function, or "off," in the usual sense of splitting, depends on the use to which it is put by the self and the self in relation to the other. As Bollas (Chapter 5) suggests, each requires separate study. Any such hypertrophy of mind is, as Winnicott, Ferenczi, and the contributors to this volume note, intended to protect a breaking heart or a flagging will. It comes about when someone, out of deprivation, deprecation, or some other reason, employs his or her mind in lieu of another object.

And once the object mind is in place, it takes on a life of its own. Its care and tending go beyond concerns with cultivation and nourishment. The possessors of such minds fear for its corruption by junk, claptrap, cants, dissimulation, and, above all, lies. Whether they defend it with a command of facts, with reason or logic, or with intuitive devices, their intent is to see through the beguiling apparitions and mirages with which they feel themselves confronted. They take misrepresentations seriously and personally; nothing is more unforgivable than an attempt at blandishment. Nothing, correspondingly, is more precious than simple candor. People like these tend to like children and other innocents. They like art that is sincere, crafts that are authentic, fields of study that do not admit to temporization, such as science or mathematics, but even in these they are suspicious of received truths, of established procedures. These last induce temptations toward dependency, to simple trust, even illusion—and such enticements to naive belief are the songs of Circe. Envy between the minds is inevitable insofar as each is greedy for attributes and dominion.

Bollas has vividly portrayed here and elsewhere (1992) the somewhat forlorn status of the subject mind when the object mind too much prevails. The subject mind—sometimes misleadingly referred to as "the" unconscious—must then quest for, create, or both, objective correlatives through which it can become realized, transformed, or transformative. Stewart refers to Bion's paper on thinking, which says that there can be an excess of alpha-function. In my own language, which also follows Bion's, preconceptions must meet with experiences so that they can evolve into realizations concerning hope and desire. Bollas's patient, Helmut, needed these; he had to find further realizations for both his parents so that they, and he with them, could come back from Splitsville. Referring to the Corrigan and Gordon chapter, he notes how the mind in his Helmut, like that in their Simon, takes a spurt of growth—"premature mental development"—when the other people in the child's life have somehow become pruned. My patient illustrates much the same thing.

Still, as is so often the case, the crux of the question is why some people take one path, others another. It may be of some importance to make a distinction between the precocity of mental function and the precocity of mind. The wise child is a child who uses his mind precociously. But there is also a precocious development of the object mind, which compensates for maternal density. When the infant cannot use the other as an object mind, either because what the infant experiences is too painful and disturbing for the other to endure or because the other is otherwise preoccupied, the lack seems to stimulate the rapid development of alpha-function and the object mind. In Bion's terms, there are simply too many thoughts to be thought for thinking not to have to snap to attention—too much ham and cheese. As I note in the prologue to my collected papers (Boris 1994a), my father's willingness to make up stories out of elements I provided was more than pleasant and congenial (aspects of us as a COUPLE); it was helpful in easing my precocity.

The patient to whom I referred came to see me when in his late twenties, remained for eight years, then briefly returned for a while two or three years later to tell me of an adventure the significance to him of which he felt, based on our work together, only I could truly appreciate.

I note as I choose this way of reintroducing my patient that it features time. "Time out of mind" is a phrase that I think of. And the way I began was with a story that is among other things, about time and looking. My patient was himself fond of looking, fonder even than I. He liked looking at naked women in the flesh, in photos, and in movies. So passionate was his love of looking that he had trained himself to be able to look while his gaze was apparently focused elsewhere. As a further aid to looking without being seen to look, he tried to make himself not much to look at. He wore seemingly nondescript versions of the standard university uniform, made his face bland and vague, and used enough of a stutter to make people want to look away.

Looking is a preferred mode of perception in the calculated construction of the subject mind by the object mind because seeing is a distal sense and more subject than the others to autonomous control. He can look even when someone moves out of range of the more proximate senses. And he can *not* look, if it suits him, even close up when it is difficult not to hear, smell, touch, or even perhaps taste. He can look without being seen to look, or calculate what people see of him. If his intellect is such as to permit him to look within, quarks and colors dance for him. Eigen (Chapter 6) makes the point that, "Prematurity is linked with a kind of visual precocity."

Nondescript my patient might seem to be, but a closer look would reveal the clothing of a connoisseur—the scuffed shoes from L. L. Bean, the worn jeans from Levi-Strauss, cashmere sweaters perfectly articulated with the shabby jackets of the original Harris tweed. The idea seemed to be: "But when they took another look . . ." A bad haircut could devastate him for a month.

Safe from barbers and vases, at the center, at the core, was his mind. And a very good mind it was. I personally delighted in it. I loved the way it worked. I envied it. My patient was a devoté of Kant and Wittgenstein. In the Tractatus, Wittgenstein (in Byatt 1965) describes the net—a picture of the way concepts, ideas, thoughts, connections of thought can be used. He asks us to imagine a surface irregularly white and black. By covering it with a fine mesh net of tiny squares, each square can be accounted as black or white.

> In this way I shall have brought the description of the surface to a unified form. This form is arbitrary because I could have applied with equal success a net of triangular or hexagonal mesh. . . . Laws like the law of causation, etc., treat of the network and not of what the network describes.[4] [p. 16]

4. I am indebted to A. S. Byatt's (1965) work on Iris Murdoch's early novels for this and other consideration of "degrees of freedom."

But what does the network describe except what the network describes? My patient agreed that the forms are arbitrary; he wanted to be sure that I knew that, too. He felt his life changed when he came to understand Einstein's theory of general relativity. He found my interpretations of considerable interest and occasional use. But he often seemed to try to understand what laws of causation lay within them rather than to put them directly to use. He wanted to work out the equations and algorithms for himself. He didn't debate or scoff at my interpretations as clever people do in the way of resistance. Rather the reverse: he wished, often for reason, they could be better derived and applied.

He had a Bionian sort of mind, and in one line of my transference fantasies I imagined myself introducing him to Bion's writings, for these I felt sure would, more than my own, have appealed and applied. I would very much have liked to discover what he would do with Bion's suppositions and how he might take them further.

Because his mind was his proudest possession, it too was worn lightly, was shabby genteel. Though I believe he might have done original work in science or mathematics, he chose instead to teach. I had no doubt that his mind partly stood in for his penis, and that in teaching he was making a particular use of it. But, as usual, why *that* symbol for that object and process?

In his case, mind was not only penis, but all the forerunners of the penis. It was the maternal breast, the thumb and pacifier, it was the hand with its prehensile thumb, it was the magic lantern, and the body, and then eventually the dick. Such is the virtuosity of the mind that when used this way, it does not really have to outgrow its earlier metamorphoses; they do not have to become vestigial. The mind accretes meaning and function; it evolves in ways that children love—it becomes this and that and that and that. Moreover the nature of the mind is such that it doesn't reduce to its constituents. It is process and content; it is container and contained. It is subject and object, perceiver and perceived. It is Narcissus and mirror. The sheer ease and fluidity of mind make it a perfect autistic object, the pre-Teddy to turn to for amusement, solace, sentience. In my patient's case, it didn't (in a certain sense) hurt that his mother admired his intelligence.

He was his mother's eldest child; she had him tested and enrolled in Mensa; one could guess that his mind functioned as her dick, too. Then came another boy when he was less than 2; this boy became an exceptional athlete. Then several years later came a girl; it would take a long struggle before it was clear what the sister would become.

My patient had nothing nice to say about his mother, though sometimes later on, he would say doubtfully that she tried. He thought her banal and plastic, full of clichés and predictable, obvious, shallow, and superficial. She seemed absolutely to have no breasts. For months on end he would not pick up his answering machine for fear of hearing her voice. His particular despair was that, instead of saying she wanted to talk with him or even remonstrating with him about his distance, she would give a pretext for why she was calling. There was no doubt that this drove him almost crazy. And no doubt that each time he was outraged afresh. He thought of killing her. But killing himself in front of her, by these means to show her what she was doing to him, always seemed more befitting. With his death he could stop the outrage; but he wanted also to teach the lesson, and I think the reason he didn't kill himself was that he feared she wouldn't get it even then.

He rather liked his father, though he felt there was, over the years, less and less to say. There had been good times when they actually worked on things together. His father was inventive and adept at electronics. Later, when in analysis, my patient bought an old car, he and his father worked on it together. Over the years the father became depressed and suicidal (for which my patient blamed his mother) and went on antidepressants, which made him brittle and false. My patient felt about him at those times the way people feel when chalk squeals on a slate. To hear his father, so obviously depressed, speak so cheerfully and facilely also nearly drove him crazy. He longed for one of his father's old temper outbursts, the way we long for a rainstorm to break a still, humid afternoon.

Of course he missed his parents tremendously—the mother behind the cunning careful pretexts, the father behind the cheerful drug-induced mask. But did he want his mother to see his despair and have a change of heart? Or was it her mind he was after: did he want a change in that? In time I analyzed the gesture of killing himself in front of his mother as his creation of the *Pietà*—the Michelangelo, in which mother and son can be confused with Dante and Beatrice or Paolo and Francesca. What if he could cry out, "Please, Mother, love me, tend me!" and she could and would? This is what I meant earlier when I said that, once established, mind takes on a life of its own. Much as he yearned for the tenderness she might afford him, there was a deep way in which he had given up on that. When he felt with his mind, his mind felt only insult and outrage. He wanted now a meeting of the minds. He was passionately concerned that she know not only what she was doing but what she had and hadn't done to him. In fact, he believed that she did know—it was just that she refused to acknowledge it. This refusal to acknowledge it seemed to him infinitely cruel and perverse. What she had done to him was not to make him feel that it was all right for him to be alive. She had given him birth, but she had not given him life. He was left, he felt, somehow twisting in the wind, like a Beckett character. It was as if there were a permission receptor pulsing darkly in the night that he hadn't been plugged into. It required of him a constant effort of will to keep on going. Such willfulness derives from the will to live. When that will is secure and certain, one doesn't find such willfulness. It attains what Eigen (Chapter 6), following Lacan, refers to as its exacerbated violence when that will cannot find the circumstances under which it can "let be."

Like many clever people, my patient envied simplicity; he envied a little boy whose sessions sometimes followed his—this youngster arrived with a clatter of enthusiasm that permeated the soundproofing. He imagined this child as if at a parental knee, eagerly confiding, avidly taking in. In this context he despised his own paranoia. He keenly felt how little he could do this. His thoughts on the subject were, he felt, captured in memories of Musical Chairs, one of the games organized by his parents for the children's birthday parties. That there was one chair too few and that he would run out of what I told him Anthony Powell called "the music of time" drove him to a frenzy. He felt that the implication that he would have to fight, which meant kill, to get his was simply much too much for him. He believed that anyone could easily see that this precisely was what he could not do. The game, he felt, cruelly mocked and exposed that inability.

He would not accept that his parents might have been insensitive; they were, to his mind, reminding him of his peculiar condition in life. That they knew, that they had reason to know, that he would have known in their place, that he knew them without having to be told, that finally he knew them better perhaps than they knew themselves—these were the axioms of his existence. In the first chapter of this volume Corrigan and Gordon raise the question of whether intelligence predisposes to certain sorts of dilemmas. There is probably something to intelligence (and imagination) that unprotects the mind—one *cannot but* discern too much—making one's recourse either an increase in his or her isolation or a vitiation of his or her ego (the disestablishment that Bollas discusses under "confusional states"). When, despite his mighty efforts to insulate himself, my patient came into contact with his father's garrulous antidepressant cheerfulness or his mother's studiously contrived but never admitted pretexts for seeing him, he was in the position of the man who knew too much for his need to know and, worse, couldn't unknow it. He felt, then and still, insult and outrage. In the consulting room at these moments he would smash and hurl the tissue box, roaring and whimpering like an animal in a trap. Sometimes he would bite deeply into his hand or wrist, as if to bite his way free.

This theme—the exploitation of his inability to fight back—was everywhere. Early on, before I saw its proportions, I attached some significance to an incident in which, driven beyond his ability not to mind, or at least not to show he minded, his brother's teasing, he whirled on the boy (who was pursuing him up the stairs) and knocked him flying such that he broke his arm in the fall. Pres-

ently I saw that though he was, of course, frightened by the unexpected (and pleasing) consequences of his self-assertion, the event
became monitory for an already well-established disposition toward
moral helplessness in the face of the demands of others: "They know
what it does to me and they do it anyway!" He felt himself alone.
He knew, knew all too well, his potential for harm—the fear of which
Coltart (Chapter 2) rightly considers absolutely basic: what sort of
arrogance was there in others that enabled them not to know theirs?

What he knew became an accretion in direct proportion to the
indifference on the part of others either to know or to use what
they knew about the consequences of their acts. His—what shall I
call it, sensibility? fascination? percipience? sensitivity? produced
an overabundance of knowledge that at times reached staggering
proportions. Is the sin in the deed; was the oedipal crime in what
the little family did or in their know-it-all, know-nothing attitudes
toward knowing? Not-so-simple Simon asks, "How are we to understand all of this?" The famous refrain from Watergate—who knew
what and when did he know it?—goes not to the crime but the cover-
up, not to the question of who *did* what, but who knew and pretended not to know. This was on its way to again becoming the case
when the vases appeared in front of the paintings. Knowing becomes
radioactive. How envious the man or woman who knows too much
can feel of those who say, "Know? Know what?" There was a period in my patient's life when he committed certain sexual misdeeds
without knowing or caring. Then he bit the apple, or, as he felt it,
the apple bit him. He lived ever since in shame and horror and in
an effort at reparation.

When, in alluding to the incident of the vases, I said my patient
took a certain pity on me, I meant by talking to me he was allowing
for the possibility that I might not have known both what I did and
what my ignorance of my deed did to him. He offered, furthermore,
that I was not altogether bloody minded, but educable (what the
patient hears, after all, is not so much what one has to say but what
one has in mind in saying it). But it was not enough for him simply
to tell me his reaction to their appearance; he felt he had to instill
in me an inclination to see that my language of the vases and flow-

ers was insinuating something in him as a result of something out of control in me. Only if I assimilated and held his juxtaposition of the vases to my picture of what I was doing and why could he once more unknow what he knew both about the two-position (preoedipal) universe and about my putative impatience: Did *he* have to know *both* our minds? By nodding he signified he knew I would be looking to see how he had taken what I said. He was also setting me an example about taking-in and acknowledging.

My patient's mother was, according to my patient, a diligent student of child development. She always seemed to know what phase and stage he was in and what sort of personality type he was, and hence what his words expressed and his behavior really meant. She did not need to be told. Wherever he went, her idea of him had preceded him. She was unsurprisable. She was prepossessed. He could not, he felt, come alive in her mind, to grow and develop in that ozone-fresh air of mild astonishment that most of us feel on contemplating the particularities of another human being. He could not, that is, gain access to her mind except insofar as he had already been there in her nosology.

I would seem to be writing of projective identification and the mother's and father's capacity for reverie and surmise, but I am trying also to speak of the problem many children have when their parents understand them "only too well"—that is, in a way unconnected with the child's own communicative efforts. (This, too, can happen in analysis when the analyst knows without having to be shown and told and made to realize. And sometimes, when the analyst is trying to get good at something, the analysis is like this: the patient illustrates the point, proves the theory.) Such knowingness creates a superfluity; knowledge becomes a drug on the market and mind has to become more concerned with the destruction of knowledge than with its generation and use. The perspicacious capacity to mimic (the opposite of the game Simon Says) characteristic of Ferenczi's (1933) Wise Child detaches the meaning of the act from its performance. T. S. Eliot refers to it as "the Shadow" that falls as if between conception and the reality, the intent and the realization. But the destruction of significance that this detach-

ment leaves represents a perspicuous hollow agape with susceptibility to influences. One senses this in Corrigan and Gordon's little
patient (Chapter 4) and his attempt to "marker" everything that
might otherwise mark him with exactly such susceptibility; beware
of tracks lest they become two-way. What Ferenczi calls the traumatic trance and Bion (1970) referring to the powers of the group
mentality over the individual sensibility, called the "numbing sense
of reality" (p. 149)[5] represents precisely such openness to influence—
to selection. This is a response to the quantity and quality (e.g.,
preemptive) of the projective identifications to which the child has
been exposed. Beware the vases.

In the creation of mind, the environment imbues only some of
the waiting potentia with meaning and function. Many are called,
few are chosen. But choice in this sense requires negotiation. Me?
Yes, you. *Me?* Yes, *you*! In this feedback loop, a sort of reciprocal
propagation takes place, which will in time come to amalgamate
with ideas of reproductive procreation. The infant or child who
cannot sire or spawn his or her experiences in the mind of another
is not merely deprived of seeing himself in a mental mirror; he comes
to doubt, whether he is meant to flourish and procreate his own
kind. Consider (as I read it) Helmut's "I scream van."

My patient's envy of his mother for herself seeming to possess,
but neither sharing nor yielding, the right to live, flourish, and
propagate was such as to drive him into identifications in which, at
the same time as he attempted to make her qualities his own (identify with her projections), he tried not to give her their authorship.
Like other of the patients mentioned in this volume, he was not
aware, was horrified to discover, how his sense of rightness aped
hers. Of Dolores, Eigen (Chapter 6) writes: "Buried at the heart of
openness was, ironically, a moralistic and judgmental element that
made life unbearable." He could stand to know as much about her
and as little of her as she him.

---

5. Bion elaborates: "The analyst feels that he is being manipulated so as to be playing a
role in some one else's phantasy—or he would do so if it were not . . . for a temporary loss
of insight, a sense of experiencing strong emotions and at the same time a belief that their
existence is adequately justified by the objective situation."

This was an envious thing to do, a riposte to what he felt she was fostering in him with her projective identifications. This left this very bright boy with a mind that was supposed to be and do what his mother was able to be and do, and be it and do it better than she—so much better than she, indeed, that what she was and did wasn't even in the picture. When the relationship becomes internalized, it retains its mutually envious nature. He strove to rise above this with his object mind, and a strain it was; where she seemed closed and unreceptive, he became a kind of Holden Caulfield, open to relativism and attuned as catcher of children. Often my interpretations, such as they were, came back from him apter and more subtle than anything I could recall saying.

Before retiring for the night, my patient's mother made a habit of checking on the children and selecting their clothes for the next day. I think one night he realized this and it took him by surprise. As a result he schooled himself to stay awake, no matter the lateness of the hour. When she approached his bed he play-acted at almost awakening, so that she would sit at the edge of his bed and stroke him back to sleep. But this was a paradox of contact. If he subsided and pretended sleep, she would leave. If he awoke, she would get up from sitting on the side of his bed. As he grew older, he saw that he must affect great restlessness, and by rolling this way and that, but more that way than this (Humbert Humbert had nothing on my patient), he could cop what sensations he could from his mother's abutting presence. But none of this could be known; she mustn't know what ideas he had or she would declare, Puberty! . . . and all would be lost. His wish for physical access expressed his failure to achieve mental access. How interesting of her also to be asleep.

In his teens, he had a girlfriend who shared with him strong intellectual, emotional, and sexual ties. But much as he enjoyed their kissing and petting, the exhilarating moments were for him the sudden espying of her breast reflected in the mirror or seeing her from an oblique angle. These arresting moments became, therefore, moments not to share so much as to harvest. They became the stuff of his drawings, in which he would put her in all kinds of perspectives, and his fantasies, where his great admiration for Busby Berkeley supplied instruction. To them he added other stolen moments, glimpses of other girls standing before him or seen through windows in the night. Around this, he arranged a compendium, formed an archive. He also increased his collection of magazines. In a sense they reached their apogee when he would dress in bits of her and his mother's clothes and masturbate into the mirror.

"What you see in them, I don't know," his mother would say of his collection of *Playboys*. "Of course she was completely flat-chested," he said when relating this. He meant always to say this with disdain, but more often than not he spoke with awe. He might also have meant was that her mind was completely flat-chested, too. As is common, he found the merging of the pictured scene with the remembered or hoped-for one particularly engaging. You will hear here an echo of my own putative movement from the two-dimensional to the three-dimensional; his intent had been to move decisively in the other direction. He hoped to replace the 3-D image with something flatter. This had reference to his mother's flat bosom; but it also expressed his envy of the original dimensional object that was capable of inflicting so much pleasure, inviting so much pain. It was as if he domesticated it. Where others ravished rosebuds, he pressed them dry between the pages of his imagination. He had them on tap day or night. Any woman who frustrated him during the other hours of the day had, little did she know, a naked counterpart in the archive. "No one, but no one escapes the Spanish Inquisition," I once told him, quoting a line from the Monty Python series he adored. But no woman who pleased him escaped either.

One day his girlfriend provided him one of those moments that seem to define something. They had been apart the first year of college, and one bright evening of summer they reunited. They talked well into the night, and as had become their way, she took over. But this time she apparently took over with dash. First she tied his hands and legs to the bedposts. Then stripping him naked, she stood above him on the bed and did a strip tease. And then— and here is the surpassing moment of what may have been a well and truly received projective identification—standing astride him, she masturbated. Naked, supine, helpless, guiltless, the man-baby excited this woman until (presumably) she couldn't stand it anymore. "Of course she knew what it would do to you and she did it anyway," I said many months later. He perceived my meaning instantly.

"And here we have, yes, the mother of this little family." My patient, as a boy with microphone in hand, was broadcasting live the events of the day. Why couldn't he have just let them be and gone about one or another of the thousand and one hobbies and projects that filled his afternoons and evenings? He designed games, solved math and logic problems, built and unbuilt electronic devices.

There was in this broadcasting live something more than an attempt to energize or make contact, something more than reparation. There was the intermediation of the self—the man who made her what she is today, folks. This same psychology is at work, according to Bion (1970), in the mentality of the liar, who also, he feels, tries to interpose himself between things as they are and the direct access of the observer.

The creative and generous side of this is to discern something in what otherwise looks like chaos or dishabille—or death; my patient had a flair for this. As at once a Holden Caulfield and a fine and dedicated teacher, his stock in trade was to see what his student's incorrect answers were correct answers to. By reconstructing what the student was trying to do, he could show him or her the methods in their mistakes. (For this same reason, he liked analysis—at least insofar as he felt that rather than attacking his mind or imposing my interpretations or my keys to his puzzles, I contented myself with revealing the method and motives for his madness. We could dispute later whether the madness was a feature or a flaw.) One evening at a party, he saw that a woman, an old friend, had a hole in her underwear. She was bright, literary, artistic, pretty—that he knew and had known; but tonight she had a hole in her undies. He felt very tenderly toward her, but she wasn't having any of it (possibly she didn't know about her panties, or know that he knew; possibly she didn't care or find it expressive).

There is something rather nuanced in this interplay between affectation and spontaneity, between arrogance and deference, be-

tween exhibitionism and revelation—just to take two or three examples. Did he want to discover the hole in the student's answers
or that there was more to the hole than the student knew? I knew
how much he wanted to heal his mother and father; I knew how he
hated them.

I thought his creations ingenious, sufficiently so that for a while
it did not strike me that rich though they were in intellect and fantasy, they lacked imagination. They had the nature of a collage,
intricate and engaging, but not lovely the way, say, a patchwork quilt
is, when the object of the latter is to preserve in nostalgic contexts
each piece in the surround of the others. It is the difference perhaps between the impulse of the collector and that of the conserva-
tor. Fantasy animates things with the heavy breathings of passion;
people and events are constrained to suit one's wishes for access,
triumph, or revenge. Imagination transports things to greater, not
lesser possibility. Both creativity and fantasy require ingenuity, the
one to expand possibility the other to confine it. "Love," writes Iris
Murdoch, "is the extremely difficult realization that something other
than one's self is not merely actual but real." Reality, she adds "is
something we are constantly and overwhelmingly tempted to deform
by fantasy" (Byatt 1965, p. 17).

He left the party with another woman (she asked him to drive
her home) and he stayed with that woman for years. She did not
dress well but was well dressed always. There was from the first no
doubt that this woman was for him a double for his mother. There
was to my mind very little doubt that this woman also symbolized
death. While he was with her he could not do other than she wanted
or what he thought she wanted, which was to stay and serve. As she
was not fond of intercourse, and shy about his penis generally, their
lovemaking consisted each evening of hours of cunnilingus. I called
what he was doing penile servitude, and he agreed. It fitted the
perennial motif: *She knows what it does to me and she does it anyway.* It was necessary to him to believe that people know whereof
they do.

To the classic constituents of bringing the erotic impulse into
play in the sexual act was added my patient's hatred of asking—of

wanting. Wanting was degrading and he would no more be found wanting than She or He or I. Out of a respect for the quid pro quo, he spared others the difficulty in asking (revealing) what he assumed they must feel too. Instead he used his intelligence and his capacity to put himself in others' shoes and think of what in any given circumstance they must be needing or wanting. I sometimes spoke of a baby who could not bear to desire linked up to a mother who could only want with pretexts and imagined how precarious the conjunctions necessary to life might become.

Deeply embedded in his complex was his idea that unless he could somehow change her mind she was going to enslave and use him up. This fate he hoped to escape through his servitude and by bringing her to her senses. If he could not ask for what he wanted, she must come to see it for herself, as his girlfriend did when she stood astride him and let him incite her to shameless excitement and pleasure. Neither said a word. But the essential point, to him, was that he was willing to cultivate his capacity for vicarious intuition (that often brings its possessor such pain) and responsible enough to use it in someone's behalf.

Elsewhere (1993) I have discussed the singular importance of the vicarious mind and its origins in the PAIR mentality. The vicarious mind whose métier is sharing through identification—there go I—is to an extent unappreciated in the literature, which tends to confine itself to the rather pedestrian issue of empathy, of "I know how you feel; I've felt that way myself." The imagination, however, is bigger than that, more capable of losing itself. The sympathetically attuned mind is capable of losing itself in the sensuous sight and sounds of the ulterior world and by process of even more imaginative sympathies, it is capable of intuiting the pure form of Platonic principles out of which phenomena comport themselves—whether these involve physics or metaphysics. (Bertrand Russell makes the point that such PAIR or vicarious love is a one-way love because the universe of form and function, like Spinoza's God, does not love in return.) The Wittegensteinian net is woven exceedingly fine *and of mesh by no means obvious to the surveyor.* The idiot savants know it, for example, in the nature and reason of the patterning of numbers, sounds, or images, the mystic in the tremors of meaning which nebulae evoke.

When will, egotism, and belief and disbelief are suspended there arises, or more accurately re-arises, in the one a profound attunement to the figuring forth of the other. This is the subject mind, unhindered, at work. This aspect of mind introjectively identifies, drawing the semaphores of social existence deep into the reciprocating elements of the individual's mentality. This is normative for the members of a PAIR; it makes it possible to communicate without consciousness and verbal language. (If the PAIR is what the PAIR does, this is what the PAIR is.) This bent toward what, after Keats, I have called "unheard melodies" is also what creates the susceptibility to the projections and projective identifications transmitted with various degrees of urgency and specificity by the group. It is what gives us the capacity to receive and transmit projective identifications. (Transferences and countertransferences occur in the COUPLE.) Under certain circumstances attunement becomes accommodation, even submission. Like Coltart's and Stewart's patients,[6] my patient felt deeply frightened of his gullibility. He, for example, felt that to surmise was to obey. He didn't need to be told. "Unheard melodies" sometimes played ditties, sometimes tattoos in his subject mind.[7]

The PAIR and the COUPLE are coterminous; when there is too little of either, the other becomes distended and engorged. When the soma and its libidinal life are suppressed, the mind turns sadosexual; when the mind is overtaxed, the body turns psychosomatic or, in Bion's phrase, "soma-psychotic." My patient, as I've said, did not like to want; it is also true that he did not like to have to speak of what he

---

6. Coltart's limericks, I think, expressed her resolve not to be taken in by the capital-M mind which was ready to pronounce on her existence in his absence. Insomnia, too, has the meaning of succumbing to belief. Stewart's is afraid of being taken in by his kindness.
7. The tedious tenacious arguments that Helmut had with his suicidal mother could only be interrupted by a fresh voice from the group—Bollas's own. Bollas's steadfast conviction that Helmut could be informed by his own banished mind provided new leadership to the Helmut PAIR, especially as Bollas appeared able to sustain attack without having, like Sphinx in *Oedipus Rex*, to end his life in the face of being discovered.

wanted. To speak represented to him a failure of communication through intimation. Vases spoke more eloquently than words. There is a line of analytic thought that regards such an "ascendancy" of mind as reaction formation. This line goes from my patient's servitude to women to its opposite—and has him reversing role and projecting impulse, such that what he fears is what in other circumstances he would sadistically impose. There is another line of interpretation that would account for his fear of dying as a screen for the fear of killing the other through his intemperate use of him or her—a not altogether secure foothold upon the Winnicottian Age of Concern.

In fact, the directional arrow is likely to be fluid and dependent on where subject and object are standing when the reading is taken. This is especially the circumstance where the vicarious mind is prominent. Vicarious knowledge leaps categories, permeates boundaries. It is interactionalistic. What happens on one side of the equation is bound to what happens on the other.

Indeed, the equation itself is jittery. There is a butterfly of chaos residing somewhere within it. I think it might be true to say that my patient suffered from the archaic superego forcing a retreat from natural dispositions, but it is not so clear whose this superego was or whether it was an introject or a self-consuming fire that didn't get damped. Sometimes I wondered if his violence wasn't a reaction to his reaction formations. In any case, I began to think that he had a feeling prior to any other, namely that he didn't have any rights. By this I mean not the right to compete and take his own position at the expense of others, but the right to live, flourish, and procreate at all. I began to think that his subject mind and object mind were the result of a large number of prior attempts to come into being, attempts that didn't make the cut.

Freud wanted us to know about the Oedipus complex, in which castration anxiety figures so prominently. Thus his basic version of the unconscious knows nothing about death and dying. His equation of death and castration is meant to read one way. But while I think that may be very well the case for the COUPLE, it is not true of the mentality of the PAIR.[8] As I indicated, in the mentality of the COUPLE, three makes a triangle, linked by rivalries; in the PAIR, three makes for a group, bound together by identifications. The question for the group is who's in and who's out—who lives and who dies—and the attitude required is an agreement to abide by the rules. In the group the important question of survival is the group's (in essence, the species) and not the individual's. The individual in his subject mind goes along with this; it is part of his nature both that he subject himself to selection and that he not think even once about it.

In his servitude that was principally but not exclusively sexual, my patient's plotline was a hapless submission to breakdown and death. Two of his dreams expressed this succinctly. In one he and I are sitting cozily on a couch in front of a fire. Then someone joins us, then another and another. Making room each time, he falls off the end of the couch. In another, he is in his car, which is speeding wildly out of control in an absence of brakes. Knowing that it will crash, he jams the gear into reverse, whereupon the car halts. But all its machinery has come into the passenger compartment impaling him. It is plain that he is now immobilized and will soon die. Even in the manifest content one can see the themes of the musical chairs of childhood recollection and the immobilization of his experience with the lover who tied him down. What he wanted was to turn these stories into a voluptuous surrender to sex. What he found—found again and again—was a time-consuming enslavement to someone else's essentially solitary sexual proclivities, for which the only real pleasure (discounting that gained by keeping her from someone else) was the hope that minds would change. When he was free to be by himself, he looked up this woman, as he routinely did others, in his archive. Oh, the things he had her do for him, and she didn't even know it. Was

---

8. Kristeva (1987) gives an interesting reading of Freud's earlier and later positions on this question. Referring to the Freud post-1925, she writes: "Does this mean that dread of dying—which henceforth is not summed up in castration fear but includes it and adds it to the wounding and perhaps even the loss of integrity of the body and the self—finds its representations in formations that are called 'transconscious' in the imaginary constructions of the split subject, according to Lacan?" She replies: "Doubtless so" (pp. 26–27).

he protecting these women from his gross nature, or was he depriving them of being needed and wanted?

In both events, my patient, as I said, was fleeing ultimacy. He had holed up. He pulled the shades and closed the drapes and worked only by lamplight. The subject mind is timeless. Within it, things rise and fall, come and go; but by providing the net through which they are apprehended, the object mind contains these. When I first met him, he wore his watch set to British time; now he didn't wear a watch at all.

> The clock is Shandy's first symbol. Under its influence he is conceived and his misfortunes begin, which are one and the same with this emblem of time. Death is hidden in clocks, as Belli said; and the unhappiness of individual life, of this fragment, of this divided, disunited thing, devoid of wholeness: death, which is time, the time of individuation, of separation, the abstract time that rolls toward its end. Tristram Shandy does not want to be born, because he does not want to die. Every means and every weapon is valid to save oneself from death and time. If a straight line is the shortest distance between two fated and inevitable points, digressions will lengthen it; and if these digressions become so complex, so tangled and tortuous, so rapid as to hide their own tracks, who knows—perhaps death may not find us, perhaps time will lose its way, and perhaps we ourselves can remain concealed in our shifting hiding places. [Calvino 1988, p. 47]

Perhaps this hiding can evolve into the kind of compulsive doubting, Descartes's alter ego, in Phillips's recounting, elaborated for himself. The premature surmise that one is not among those meant to live, of course, puts one's very existence in doubt. It is akin to a beta-element, and requires either generous dollops of reassurance or a lot of mental alpha work to be managed. I agree with Bollas (1992) and Piontelli (1988), Osterweil (1990), and Mitrani (1994) that the question arises *in utero* when the intimations are likely to be little more than chemical innundations. But the dread these intimations conduce can hardly be overestimated. No wonder the autistic enclaves to which Tustinian neonates gravitate are meant to

be impermeable! My patient's habit of working around the clock in
lamplight (he loathed fluorescent overhead lighting) conjuring, like
the younger Faust, with his formulas and formulations matters that
had thus far escaped cognitive rendering was his solution: Mind
could catch death in its net and make it alpha; that net could be
studied and refined by careful analysis including psychoanalysis. As
Phillips puts it apropos Descartes, "Mind, intelligence, intellect,
reason; words born of necessity, *insuring a future*" (emphasis is my
own). For the great thing about the mind-net is so long as it was
catching death, death is not, like some perverse fisher of men, catching one.

The terrible irony in this is that, as with so many forms of evasion, in fleeing what he feared my patient became the prisoner of
his sanctuary.[9] Feeling that with mind he could make those imperious efforts of the will on which he felt his life depended, he feared
the loss of his mind as others might of their lives. As light discovers
dark and dark light, hot–cold, hard–soft, so life does death and death
life: You can't think space without thinking time: you can't think
one without the other. Hence my remark to him, apropos the vases,
about what he feared from me. This man was among a number of
other patients who were nudging me into thinking about the question of selection, which later I began to feel able to formulate.

From this, you will have surmised that the only thing my patient
really asked of me was an abeyance of time. He hated that we should
end on time. But more than that, he craved marathon sessions. His
mind, he told me, did not work in segments. He went on to say that
what I am calling the object mind so intruded on the subject mind
that he could not, to his satisfaction, lose himself in free association for all that we were meeting five times each week. I had a great
deal of internal difficulty with this: I thought that he had every right
to try marathon sessions, and I also thought that the request would

---

9. There is a scene in a Michael Innes novel, *The Case of the Journeying Boy* (1909), in
which the terrified boy barely escapes his pursuers; he is safe at last in a bus that is taking
him away from Oxford, and safer still, he feels, to be seated next to a woman of the cloth.
Until, that is, he sees, as the nun's hands are removed from the sleeves of her habit, the
dark wiry hair on "her" fingers.

yield value if subjected to analysis. It was not as if he was unable to experience his experience and speak of it, but I also knew that there was a stream of madness of which he was very chary. If it surfaced in the latter part of a session, he would stifle it. For better or worse, thinking that this paramount issue between us would yield much to analysis, I asked him, finally, if he could postpone the question for a while, so we could examine his feelings. He agreed; but I thought I heard tumblers falling into place as in the spinning of a combination lock: *He knows I can't do it and he makes me do it anyway.*

When he reopened the question some time later, it was too late for me, and I felt I had to tell him how illness precluded. There is no question that even as he felt sympathy for me, he felt too that once again it was too little too late, and this hardened his heart. I gradually became aware that because of what he experienced as my empathic failure he planned to make no permanent changes as a result of the analysis. And indeed, as the analysis began to conclude, my patient set about a process of reclamation. The changes he underwent in order to have a reaching analysis were authentic—and as Phillips notes, the changes the patient is required to make in order to be analyzed are in a real sense *the* changes in an analysis; but each was marked by that gossamer trail of bread crumbs by which after termination he would guide himself back. I felt more than a little sad about this variant of his perverse pietà, but I more or less consoled myself with the fact that the insights and possibilities we had together fashioned were not perishable; they would be available to him if by any chance he had a change of heart.

And there we left it. He resumed his previous occupation, reassumed his previous ways. Like Penelope, he unraveled what we wove, such that time did not pass, had not passed. His tuxedo from high school still fit; he could wear the same shoes. Our eyes were moist as we parted. Then, as I say, he came back to tell me of his change. Only I, he said, could appreciate its titanic quality. He meant appreciate and feel appreciative.

He had, while still in analysis, bought a house with a friend of long standing. For him it was an investment property, for her a place to live. Clever with things around the house, his father's son, my patient soon entered servitude and was on call day and night in every weather. Having realized a substantial paper gain on the property, my patient had, as I recalled, thought perhaps he might escape his indenture by selling his portion of it. Moreover, he could invest his profits elsewhere and once more double them. But, perhaps unsurprisingly, it was to turn out his friend had other ideas.

What my patient came back to tell me was of the struggle he went through to put the matter finally in the hands of an attorney. At first he had thought his struggle was only with her, and he tried with every contrivance he had to change her mind; he prepared reams of financial analysis, obtained statements from real estate brokers and tax experts and so on and on. He found buyers for his share and for both shares. But after a lot of this, there came a day when he suddenly understood that he was, in this argument, determinedly reclaiming his mind from my influences; and, upon this realization, he revisited his old wish to have her "acknowledge what she was doing to him," the issue of "penile servitude," and with these, additional recollections of what he himself was playing at. To this he had added a dream in which he was a woman. By the by, he told me, the woman[10] with the hole in her panties had recently resurfaced, and they were now keeping company, although he had not parted from the woman he had driven home that night long ago.

In telling me of these events he spoke of how vividly my words came back to him, how he could even, as it were, hear me voicing his insights in my characteristic manner. I felt he was telling me that he now maintained a vicarious relation of my mind with his. This idea of two minds with but a single thought is very dear within the PAIR; it inspires feelings of mystical union. (In the COUPLE narcissism is autoerotic; in the PAIR the narcissism is the bliss of unboundedness, wherein projective identifications flow freely, in both or all

---

10. The better to focus on mind, I have subordinated in this chapter the nonmind work my patient and I did, which in important respects followed the work of Anna Freud on passivity and submission. In this recounting there is the usual convergence and antagonisms of the COUPLE and the PAIR, the sensual and the nonsensuous, of hope and desire.

directions.) From this I knew, although he did not mention it, that he had also come back to see how I was faring.

At parting, accordingly, I asked him what his impressions of me were, now that we were remet. He became very serious. He had worried about my health and was very relieved, "very, very, relieved," to see me so well. Feeling he had in some sense been retrograde and remembering that for the most part I wished him well, he had come to tell me of these developments; of this much he was aware. But that he needed me to be well—had needed an alive and self-selected mind to correspond with and had come perhaps to improve my welfare by allowing me to gain a dimensional picture of him—had not been so clear to him. It surprised him, I guessed, that I still had something to tell him that he had not already filed away. But that is the way; the patients who figure in this volume continue to stimulate thought in their analysts' minds. They have at last found another mind in which to be conceived of and come alive—as if, if *you* think, therefore *I* am.

REFERENCES

Bion, W. R. (1970). *Attention and Interpretation*. New York: Basic Books.

Bollas, C. (1992). Being a Character: Psychoanalysis and Self Experience. New York: Hill and Wang.

Boris, H. N. (1993). *Passions of the Mind: Unheard Melodies: A Third Principle of Mental Functioning*. New York: New York University Press.

Boris, H. N. (1994a). *Sleights of Mind: Collected Papers*. Northvale, NJ: Jason Aronson.

—— (1994b). *Envy*. Northvale, NJ: Jason Aronson.

Byatt, A. S. (1965). *Degrees of Freedom: Early Novels of Iris Murdoch*. New York: Barnes & Noble.

Calvino, I. (1988). *Six Memos for the Next Millennium*, trans. P. Creagh. Cambridge, MA: Harvard University Press.

Damasio, A. R. (1994). *Descartes' Error: Emotion, Reason and the Human Brain*. New York: Grosset/Putnam.

Edelman, G. (1987). *Neural Darwinism*. New York: Basic Books.

Eliot, T. S. (1952). *The Complete Poems and Plays*. New York: Harcourt, Brace.

Ferenczi, S. (1933). Confusion of tongues between adults and the child. In *Final*

Contributions to the Problems and Methods of Psychoanalysis, ed. M. Balint. London: Hogarth.

Freud, S. (1925). Negation. *Standard Edition* 19:233–239.

Innes, M. (1909). *The Case of the Journeying Boy*. New York: Dodd, Mead, 1949.

James, B. (1992). *Protection*. Woodstock, VT: Countryman Press.

Kristeva, J. (1987). *Black Sun: Depression and Melancholia*, trans. L. S. Roudiez. New York: Columbia University Press.

Lorenz, K. (1965). *Evolution and Modification of Behavior*. Chicago: University of Chicago Press.

Mitrani, J. (in press). *A Framework for the Imaginary: Psychoanalytic Exploration in Primitive States of Being*. Northvale, NJ: Jason Aronson.

Ogden, T. (1994). *Subjects of Analysis*. New York: Jason Aronson.

Osterweil, E. (1990). *A Psychoanalytic Exploration of Fetal Mental Development and Its Role in the Origin of Object Relations*. Unpublished Doctoral Dissertation.

Piontelli, A. (1988). Prenatal life and birth as reflected in the analysis of a two-year-old psychotic girl. *International Review of Psycho-Analysis* 15:73–81.

Spitz, R. A. (1957). *No and Yes: On the Genesis of Human Communication*. New York: International Universities Press.

Tausk, V. (1919). On the origin of the "Influencing Machine" in schizophrenia. In *The Psycho-Analytic Reader*, ed. R. Fleiss, pp. 31–64. New York: International Universities Press,

Winnicott, D. W. (1971). *Playing and Reality*. New York: Basic Books.

10

Bracing for Disappointment and the Counterphobic Leap into the Future

Peter Shabad
Stanley S. Selinger

Many of us can remember those times in our respective school careers when one of the best students in the class would emerge from an examination and make the ritualistic declaration "I flunked" or "I did terribly." When the grades were returned, however, to no one's surprise the same student received the "A" to which he or she was accustomed. We are also familiar with those persons who cannot bear the anticipatory tension of prolonged goodbyes, who cut short their leave-taking of a loved one, even though there might be precious time remaining before departure. In clinical practice we similarly are acquainted with patients who glance at their watches three minutes before a session is scheduled to end and say, "I guess it's time to end now." There even are anecdotes in which patients have brought alarm clocks to their sessions, just so they would be able to "quit before being fired." To a greater or lesser extent, all of us say "No" to ourselves before someone else does first. We pretend to ourselves we do not want what we do not think we can get.

This process of breaking the tension, of waiting for the prover-bial ax to fall by moving more quickly toward the anticipated danger lies at the basis of the counterphobic defense. In this chapter we examine how the counterphobic process of bracing for disappointment by mentally leaping into the future is centrally implicated in the defensive aspects of human development. In those severe cases in which trauma has punctured the innocence of a child's life prematurely, development may take on a hyperstimulated, disjointed quality, as the mental bracing for future danger gives rise to a chronic sense of getting ahead of oneself.

CREATING AND FINDING

One essential constituent of healthy development lies in the capacity of the child to retain some sense of integrity or organismic wholeness as he proceeds through life. This sense of integrity also has a temporal dimension, that is, the psychosomatic unity of the child is rooted in the current moment.

It is from this rootedness in the current moment that the unfolding of organismic development is then fueled by the "spontaneous gesture" of the child. And it is the mother's meeting of that spontaneous gesture that helps establish a fluidity between wish and fulfillment. This fluidity then fosters the child's constructive illusion of what Winnicott (1960a) refers to as "continuity of being," of what Bergson (1889) refers to as a sense of duration. Here, that which the infant creates is at one with what is found.

When the baby's created image of a wished-for mother increasingly does not match the reality of the mother who is found, he must begin to cope with the times and spaces between wish and reality, between creating and finding. Rather than conceive of separation between mother and child as overtly physical, we could describe problems of the quality of attachment with more phenomenological accuracy if we view the baby's *experience* of separateness as an increasingly wide discrepancy between the wished-for mother who is created and real mother who is found.

Perhaps we can better illuminate the baby's search for the mother through the separate spaces between creating and finding, if we view it metaphorically as a journey across a desert. At first, the baby relies on the internal compass of an imagined maternal oasis to direct his quest. His hopeful conviction of reaching his destination provides the fuel of meaning necessary to his searchings.

The baby's created image of the mother is substantively nurtured whenever its approximate version is located in actuality. The child's continuous interplay of creating and finding himself through the reflected eyes of the mother contains the lonely process of searching through the spaces in between. The baby's sense of omnipotence, thus reinforced, lays the foundation for positive superstition: "What I wish for, I shall find." This positive superstition underlies the baby's innocence.

Innocence refers to the elemental conviction that one is welcome in a world that is benignly disposed toward oneself. It is a constructive illusion that enables the baby or child to place his well-being trustfully in the protective arms of a world waiting to receive and care for him. Innocence thus consists of an unconscious carefreeness that no matter what pathway one creates for one's quest, a responsive "home" of a receptive audience is to be found at the other end.

Implicit in this reliance on the receptivity and protection of others is an unconsciousness of impending threat. It is precisely this unawareness or "innocence" of evil that insulates the illusory sphere in which the child can play in a carefree way from within his going on being. The child's grounding of himself in the continuity of creating and finding provides the security necessary then to remain open to the transformational possibilities of each new moment and space between self and other. It is only gradually that his "naturalistic" buffer of innocence gives way to the development of a consciousness that still is fundamentally rooted in the psychosomatic unity of the current moment.

THE RUPTURE OF INNOCENCE

What, then, occurs when this sense of innocence is disrupted before its time? What happens when any number of impingements, frustrations, traumas, or prolonged separations prematurely evict a child from his or her private Garden of Eden? What occurs if the child continues his solitary journey across his private desert without finding the mother he seeks in due course, instead falling through the cracks between self and other and immersing for too long in the chasm of nonbeing? Here is Winnicott's (1967) description of a baby's experience of being separated from his mother as the time of her absence is extended:

> In X + Y minutes the baby has not become altered. But in X + Y + Z minutes the baby has become traumatized. . . . Trauma implies that the baby has experienced a break in life's continuity so that primitive defenses now become organized to defend against a repetition of "unthinkable anxiety" or a return to the acute confusional state that belongs to disintegration of nascent ego structure. [p. 97]

As long as the baby, toddler, or child continues to search for the created mother who is not there, he faces the prospect of encountering an unending solitude over infinitely empty expanses. When the baby's wished-for image of the mother is not supported by the experience of finding her really, the baby's image remains just that— a hallucinatory image of a maternal oasis without substance, a mirage.

As the internal compass of a hopeful image of a maternal destination breaks down into an unrealized mirage, the guiding purposefulness of searching gives way to the vague aimlessness of mental wandering. In thus losing sight of his maternal destination, the baby becomes increasingly lost and disoriented. Here the baby's experience of absence becomes increasingly flavored by a desperate anxiety and fear of not finding the mother rather than by the wish to find her. An infant's too close encounter with a prolonged unresponsive silence to his yearnings forms the basis of negative superstition: "What I wish for, I fear I will not find." Andre Green (1978) has noted: "Absence, paradoxically, may signify an imaginary presence or else unimaginable nonexistence" (p. 181). The madness of coming face to face with a mirageful silence is captured by Winnicott's notion of the "negative hallucination." Winnicott described the negative hallucination of one of his patients who reported looking in the mirror and seeing nothing. Here is Winnicott (1967) again:

> We must assume that the vast majority of babies never experience the X + Y + Z quantity of deprivation. This means that the majority of children do not carry around with them for life the knowledge from experience of having been mad. Madness here simply means a breakup of whatever may exist at the time of a personal continuity of existence. After recovery from X + Y + Z deprivation a baby has to start again permanently deprived of the root which could provide continuity with the personal beginning. [p. 97]

We might view this permanent deprivation as a traumatic puncturing of innocence. Trauma ruptures the illusory space that binds creating and finding, and which forms the core of innocence in the baby's unconscious continuity of being.

We can refer to this experience or sense of separateness as psychic loss. In contrast to the acute and overt trauma of physical loss, the experience of psychic loss derives from relatively intangible trauma extending over many years, the residual effects of which are felt only after the fact. Kris (1956) describes *strain trauma* as "the effect of long-lasting situations, which may cause traumatic effects by accumulation of frustrating tensions" (p. 73). Strain can be viewed as the ill-fated effort put forth by the child to change the environment so it better synchronizes with what the child has created in the idealized image of his wishes.

Khan (1974) uses the term *cumulative trauma* to describe "the significant points of stress and strain in the evolving mother–infant relationship." Although Khan emphasizes early mother–infant interaction as the major determinant of cumulative trauma, the concept of cumulative trauma could be extended to refer to traumas that accumulate throughout childhood, and in relation to any significant familial figure.

The traumatizing aspects of such accumulating frustrations derive from the child's everyday exposure to the constancy of a parent's characterological "faults" (to use Balint's [1968] term). The term *traumatic theme* has been used to describe the patterned imprint of

repetitive frustration that gradually emerges from the concrete interplay between the child and the most problematic aspects of the
parent's character (Shabad 1989).

A child's wish to give something good and receive something good
from a parent can be thwarted indefinitely in a variety of ways. A
parent's exploitation of a child's need to give, for example, may result
in the child's construction of a false self. Giving the "silent" treatment when angry, petty criticisms, and a parent's persistent intru-
siveness all may come to constitute traumatic themes of varying
severity. A mother's histrionic display of helplessness or a father's
explosively drunken rages, having small promises broken, being
called stupid, all may leave a cumulative imprint of trauma on the
character of the developing child. It is only in later years when as
clinicians we observe repetitive urges to undo and master the traumatic theme that the experience of psychic loss can be reconstructed.
The term *psychic loss* thus is used to complete the picture of unfulfilled longings, repetitive acting out, and the sense of incomplete
mourning often conveyed in clinical practice.

The incompleteness of the psychic loss of a physically present
parent hinders a mourning process based on the relative finality
and closure of physical loss. In the physical absence of the real
parent, hope springs eternal in the freedom of imaginative space
that the wished-for, created parent still is to be found. The idealized image of the created parent, formed during the real parent's
periodic physical absence, becomes increasingly difficult to maintain in the face of the reappearances of the same frustrating parent
who instead is the one that is found and refound, again and again.

Although the continued physical presence of the parent would
seem to contradict the child's experience of loss, on the contrary it
is precisely the physical presence of the real parent that intrudes
on the child's search for and finding of the created, wished-for
parent. After a while, from the child's viewpoint, it is not the frustratingly real parent who is the primary source of emotional torment, but his own desperate, misbegotten wish to find the ideal
restitutive parent that leaves him helplessly exposed to the cycle of
wish and disappointment.

THE COUNTERPHOBIC DEFENSE

Rather than face the "madness" of searching indefinitely in a mirror for oneself and seeing nothing, a baby adapts to the rupture of his innocence by taking the matter of his biopsychological survival into his own hands. As guardian of his own well-being, the baby must take care not to fall into the terror-laden spaces between self and other.

Similarly, sooner or later an older child consciously "gives up"; he detaches from his wishes for the idealized parent that lead only to perpetual frustration. Joffe and Sandler (1965) point out that defensive detachment occurs when the child "settles for its actual state of the self. It is a type of resignation which can be seen as an attempt to do away with the discrepancy between actual self and ideal self" (p. 409). Rather than wait indefinitely for a created, wished-for mother to materialize, the child, sensing threat to his survival, instinctively makes do and attempts to extend himself outward to meet the mother who is there.

Whereas phobia entails a retreat from impingement, counterphobia, in contrast, involves a movement toward precisely that which is most threatening or frustrating. As such, it is a means of adaptively rendering passive into active, of defending by taking the offensive. Insofar as quick, decisive action is biologically adaptive from an evolutionary viewpoint, we could say that counterphobia is a basic organismic process that has led to the "survival of the fittest." Yet even if we conclude that the chances for survival are enhanced by counterphobic defenses, we certainly cannot automatically assume that the same is true for the quality of that survival or adaptation.

The word *adaptation*, frequently employed as an insignia of functioning mental health, is a remnant of Darwin's theory of evolution. The ultimate pragmatism is one in which the organism that adjusts to an inhospitable reality is the one that survives. The very same protective mechanisms that insure survival, however, are also antithetical to the openness required for the human striving toward a meaning-filled existence. For the very same processes that enable a person to adapt to the exigencies of his environment also tear him

apart psychologically. As Winnicott noted, the natural unfolding of
the human infant can be radically diverted from its developmental
"plan" by environmental impingements.

Because the baby is unable to initiate his counterphobic movement toward impingement by crawling, walking, or running toward
the actual mother, he compensates instead through intensified
mental activity. To escape being helplessly imprisoned in a seemingly abandoned body, the baby attempts to extend himself outward
by projecting this mental activity to fill the void between self and
other, between the created, wished for mother and the found reality of the impinging mother. Winnicott (1949a) notes:

> Certain kinds of failure on the part of the mother, especially erratic
> behavior, produce over-activity of the mental functioning. Here, in
> the overgrowth of the mental function reactive to erratic mother-
> ing, we see that there can develop an opposition between mind and
> the psyche-soma, since in reaction to the abnormal environment the
> thinking of the individual begins to take over and organize the car-
> ing for the psychesoma, whereas in health it is the function of the
> environment to do this. [p. 246]

Out of the baby's mandate to care for himself emerges a pragmatic soul that must ensure that the baby avoid confronting the
blank face of annihilating nothingness at all costs, even if that means
developing a dissociative "opposition between mind and psyche-
soma." The baby's projection of a mental, disembodied extension
of himself is a desperate attempt to take up the slack for who is not
there and bring in some proof of his own real existence via an encounter with the real mother on her turf.

Simultaneous with this outward counterphobic movement to meet
the impingement head on is the child's defensively active attempt
to gain mastery or a type of ownership over the frustratingly real
mother by incorporating her into what Winnicott (1960a) calls the
"sphere of one's omnipotence." The baby imposes his own intro-
jective structure and meaning upon his experiences of frustration
by creating a false self in the image of the other's interfering, impinging needs. As an imitative replica devoted to the care of those

needs of the real mother, the false self reflects back to the baby some sense, albeit compromised, that he really exists in the world. From its vantage point in the disembodied limbo between self and other, the false self then is a projection of intensified mental activity that has the two-way purpose of being a patchwork intermediary between the real world and the baby's genuine need for realization.

From the time of the first encounter with overwhelming frustration, a counterphobic process to meet and take in the enemy is set in motion; the baby's helplessness of groping in the dark indefinitely for the mother that he has created leads to a sense of being abandoned in his body. The intensification and projection of mental activity then becomes an attempt to find an outlet to others and fill the void where the wished-for mother should be. This disembodied false self, charged with the task of overseeing the child's survival, is used to introject the image of the only mother who was found: the real one who intruded or impinged on the search for the ideal one. The baby instinctively follows, conforms to, adjusts to, imitates, and takes in the powerful "enemy" of impinging reality that is there rather than the "friend" of a hoped-for ideal that is not.

Taking on the guise of the enemy in this way, however, carries with it a heavy cost to the child's sense of integrity and continuity, as is implied in Winnicott's distinction between false self and true self. For although the false self may be a necessary "adaptation" to impingement in the most biological sense, in another, almost Faustian sense, the counterphobic construction of the false self belies a selling of one's developmental soul for the purposes of preserving one's survival.

The counterphobic movement toward impingement thus has a disintegrating effect on the child's sense of integrity in the current moment. In attempting to accommodate to frustrating reality, the child betrays himself by defensively shifting his self's center of gravity from inside to outside, from the subjective experience of helpless yearning to an identification with the more powerful negation of those yearnings, and from a rootedness in his body to an identification with vigilant, disembodied mental activity. If continually frustrated in the wish to transform the actual parent into an ideal figure, a child may later become an adolescent who, rather than experience the unbearable tension and degradation of wishes falling on deaf ears, defends against that helplessness by taking on the guise of the more powerful enemy—the hated and disillusioning behavior of the parent. Winnicott (1949a) notes that under abnormal circumstances, "One can observe a tendency for easy identification with the environmental aspect of all relationships that involve dependence, and a difficulty in identification with the dependent individual" (p. 247).

The baby compensates for who is not there by enclosing himself in a mental relationship with himself. In thus providing a home-grown mirror from the outside looking in, the baby holds himself together as if in a mental self-embrace so as not to disintegrate. In this sense, the narcissistic vehicle of self-consciousness or one's mental relationship with oneself is an involuted attempt to fill up the still silence between self and other with one's own voice.

In attempting to adapt to a parent's characterological faults, for example, the child's introjection of sadomasochistic interactions with the parent corresponding to the experiences of his traumatic theme(s) may be a relational substitute that is preferable to a more desolate, solitary encounter with a parent who seems silently and immutably unresponsive to his efforts and wishes. An actual frustrating relationship with a parent provides a more secure foundation for the development of one's identity than the longing for the actualization of an ideal relationship that never seems to materialize.

By parroting, echoing, and perpetrating on oneself the constellation of frustrating attitudes, behavior, and morality particular to one's traumatic theme(s), a child displays an ongoing, counterphobic attempt to co-opt the emotional potency of frustration by merging with its source. In this active attempt to "identify with the aggressor," to silence wishes for a longed for figure before they are silenced from without, we glimpse the fundamental core of superego processes. In this sense, the superego, formed with the mandate to watch over the survival of the ego or self, is based on the maxim that something bad is better than nothing. Like a psychic auto-immune system gone out of control, the child, through the excessive use of hypercritical, involuted mental activity, repeatedly attempts to change the impossible into the forbidden (to use Joyce McDougall's [1985] term) by gaining a type of omnipotent ownership over the traumatic experience.

In reacting to the disillusionments of the traumatic theme, the child's defensive detachment from his wishes coincides with time's ongoing indifference to his desires: without a pause of compassion, time marches forward ruthlessly. The child-turned-adolescent must either keep up and adapt to the pragmatics of growing up, or be left behind with the helplessness of unfulfilled wishes. The emotional isolation of the psychic loss experience thus may be compounded by the defensive determination to be sufficiently thick-hided so as to cope with whatever hardships "reality" may bring. Given the adolescent task of fashioning an identity fitted for the harsh rigors of adult life, we should not be surprised at the child's seeming self-betrayal in renouncing his wishes, "seeming betrayal" because in presenting the appearance of treacherously complying with the enemy by killing off his wishes, an adolescent may only be "playing dead" in a form of intrapsychic possum. By perpetually forbidding himself the expression of wishes that led only to endless disillusionment we can discern an attempt to tuck his wishes away protectively in the unconscious so that they may be resurrected for another day. Ferenczi (1909) says:

> The neurotic helps himself by taking into the ego as large as possible a part of the outer world, making it the object of unconscious phantasies. This is a kind of diluting process, by means of which he tries to mitigate the poignancy of free-floating, unsatisfied and unsatisfiable unconscious wish impulses. One might give to this process . . . the name of *Introjection* [p. 47]

THE LEAP INTO THE FUTURE

The counterphobic movement toward impingement may also be viewed from a temporal perspective, as the baby or child shifts his center of gravity from the current moment to a mental "bracing for disappointment" in the future. Human beings thus actively and dramatically introject and elaborate on their experiences of trauma, irrevocably transforming the meaning of those experiences in memory. Although the baby seeks escape from the painfully impinged upon emotionality of the body in the ethereal refuge of mental activity, those experiences of impingement must inevitably pervade the activity of thinking, which now becomes anything but an autonomous ego function. Thus, as the transformed meanings of trauma are projected onto an imaginary blank screen of the future, their residual afterimages, the transference of trauma, come to form an anticipated danger in the reflected image of the frustrating past. Once the unguardedness of innocence is ruptured, the virginal expanses of the future are sullied by the child's own projections of haunting afterimages of his experience.

Just as the dangerous future is created transferentially from the traumatized past, the cultivation of precocious mental activity, based on the dread of retraumatization, is tinged with a mistrust of all things spontaneous and unconscious. As oncoming experience is filtered through this braced mental activity, we witness the birth of character defense. Never again will this person be able to ground himself carefreely and restfully, without some primal anxiety, in the open continuous interplay of creating and finding.

The future, now and forever after, will be circumscribed, to a greater or lesser extent, by a fearful bracing for the dangers that have been transferred to its blank screen. To safeguard against the anticipated threat, the child attempts to protect his emotional nakedness so he is never caught off guard again. The anticipation of waiting to encounter the transferential afterimages of trauma infuses the child's developmental quest with a vigilant urgency, fueling it with a hyperstimulated momentum. Development, rather than resembling a graduated walking into the future, may now take the form of a running ahead.

The quickened, manic-like attempts of the hyperactive child to race ahead have a "primitive" counterphobic quality—as if it is not the immediate encounter with danger that is most dreaded, but rather the drawn-out wait for impending doom to descend. The relentless forward movement of such children is a counterphobic reaction to their own projected fears, now transformed into the silently imagined prohibitions of the future. They must rush ahead and grab before their mirage-like treasures are taken away.

Here, in the hyperactive child's frantic intrusions into the inner recesses of the therapist's desk drawers, in his frenetic searching within the closets of clinic playrooms, and in his desperate digging into sandboxes for an ever-elusive sustenance, we see a different, more ambitious side to counterphobia, something beyond the merely defensive function of foreclosing further impingement.

This becomes clear if we consider that the transference process itself has a double-edged quality. At the same time that a person transfers actual frustrating experiences that circumscribe and narrow developmental possibilities, he is also transferring idealized scenarios to the future that are designed to make up for what never took place in the past. The quickening of the counterphobic movement reflects a springing of eternal hope, a search for a longed for but ever-elusive ideal, an ideal, however, that when grasped at seems to evaporate into all-too-familiar patterns of experienced frustration.

This dual transference of the actual and ideal to the future is reflected also in two forms of repetition noted by psychoanalytic observers. Loewald (1971) has spoken of "passive repetition" and an "active re-creative repetition" and Balint (1968) has contrasted "malignant regression" and "benign regression." Whereas passive repetition and malignant regression are characterized by a compulsive participation in repetitive spirals of thought and action, active repetition and benign regression enable a person to use repetition so as to re-form psychic structure and find the sought for ideal of a "new beginning."

If the frenetic forward movement of the hyperactive child is a crude form of counterphobia, then the cultivation of precocious mental activity may be viewed as the "new, improved, technological editions" of the counterphobic process. For through the immediacy of forethought, the future is gained instantaneously. The counterphobic process of mentally leaping into the future and bracing for disappointment may be viewed as a means of subjecting the helplessness of undergoing trauma to the omnipotence of mental control. In thus turning from passive to active, the compulsion to co-opt the potency of future danger has the magical aim of cleaning up the debris of impingement so that the child may renew his unfolding path once more.

As the child flies away from the entrapping confines of his abandoned body, however, he is also mentally reinventing himself from the outside in. With the rupture of innocence and the birth of character defense, the child reconceives himself, now through the lens of mental activity. It is perhaps in this sense of the child creating himself anew mentally that we can understand Winnicott's (1967) observation that the baby "starts over" after being cut off from his beginnings.

Moreover, for the mind, born from the ashes of a dead innocence, the good-enough environment is no longer good enough. The child, with his mind in tow, must ensure that the residual debris of searching for the wished-for mother and instead finding nothing must be swept away entirely so that his path can begin again as if for the first time.

Winnicott (1949) thus notes: "The mind has a root, perhaps its most important root, in the need of the individual at the core of the self, for a perfect environment." He goes on to say, "the mind seeks a perfect environment because that would enable the individual to return to the dependent psyche-soma which forms the only place to live from. In this case, 'without mind' becomes a desired state" (p. 246).

Here we have the paradox of a person using his mind to control his internal and external environments so as to secure the renewed "perfect" sense that his survival is not at stake, enabling him finally to free himself of the cumbersome appendage of his disembodied mind. What at one time was the child's greatest ally now has become his most implacable foe. Perhaps this is one way we can understand why many so-called brilliant children burn out on the activity of thinking by the time they become adults, at which point they reach back for the mindless ordinariness of being a carefree child. In this sense, no one is immune to the homesickness of the repetition compulsion. Our adult characters are fraught with repeated symptomatic attempts to turn back the clock and find the restful grounding underlying the unconscious flow of being before it was disrupted by trauma.

THE TIME-TRAVELING MAGIC
OF MENTAL ACTIVITY

In the child's aim to begin again perfectly, as if for the first time, he enlists the time-traveling acrobatics of his mind. Through the counterphobic leap of forethought, the sequence of events and images of a child's life, past and future, may be halted and reversed. We observe from the stutterings of a first courtship, or the inhibiting effects of thought on action, that self-consciousness tends to stop the flow of a particular process in which one is participating. Consciousness brings the unpredictable dynamics of a given process under omnipotent mental control by dividing the inhibited process into discrete segments. Winnicott (1949b), in speaking of the aftermath of birth trauma, described this cataloging and counting function of mental activity.

The unfolding, indivisible flow of time is an example of a process that consciousness divides into discrete segments of past, present, and future. And Henri Bergson (1889) has noted that through the counting, quantifying function of consciousness, a notion of space is formed. Once the past is no longer viewed only as an indistinguishable aspect of the seamless, irreversible flow of lived time, but has its own discrete, reified space, it may be represented by an image such as a photograph. Once these various images of a bygone past become fixed in consciousness, they are subject to the magical beckonings of primary-process thinking in which the images of the past become grist to be manipulated into the fantasized ideals of the future.

For in the unconscious the timelessness of the circle replaces linear time. Beginnings are endings and endings are beginnings; one can go backward as easily as forward, and that which has been lost can be retrieved. By mentally locating oneself in the future, an experiential sense of distance from oneself is created, a sense of being on the outside looking in. With this shift in perspective from inside to outside, everything that was in is out and that which was out is in, and what was future is past and what was past becomes future. Shifting from body to mind and from present to future is not unlike leaping out of a bus moving in one direction and hopping on another bus moving in the opposite direction. In so doing, one may retrace one's steps to use a wrong (reenacting of trauma) to undo a wrong (trauma) and make a right (a perfect, new beginning).

The missed opportunities of the long-ago past thus may become nostalgically sentimentalized and transformed into a potential "Field of Dreams" where it becomes possible through the acrobatic magic of mental time travel to redeem old disillusionments in a utopian future. It is through the counterphobic magic of precocious thinking that a person may leap from a mortal body, necessarily anchored in one place at one time and fated to live out its one and only life, and refigure the frustrations and disillusionments of the past into a perfectible "brave new world" of the future.

It is in this "acrobatic" sense that perhaps we can look again at Michael Balint's (1968) young woman patient, whose somersault exemplified for him the notion of a benign regression to a new beginning. That somersault proved to be a clinical breakthrough for her. Not only was her somersault a successful expression of benign regression, however, but the somersault itself is at once a symbolic and physical means of standing time on its head. The patient's completion of it finally fostered the illusion, in the most concrete sense, of having created a new beginning for herself.

THE MENTAL REINVENTION OF
A BRAVE NEW WORLD

What of this mental quest for a new beginning of a perfectible brave new world then, a world animated by id magic, but shaped by the precocious thinking of what Romanyshyn (1989) calls the "mathematical"? Romanyshyn says the mathematical means the "projection in advance of the appearance of things, of precisely how those things are to appear" (p. 78).

Precocious mental activity is a characteristic means by which counterphobic defenses become manifested in an advanced technological society. It is perhaps not too farfetched to say that the hypertechnology of the modern Western world reflects a collective attempt by means of precocious mental activity to control, predict, and remake the future in the perfect image of the imperfect past. The invention of the computer, for example, manifestly reveals the counterphobic quest of its creator, the disembodied mind, a quest for a tidy cerebral universe, unsullied by the messy, "error-prone" unpredictability of unconscious feeling.

Psychoanalysis, characterized as it is by the rational dissection of unconscious experience into its constituent parts, may be viewed as a counterphobically motivated technology of the human mind specifically designed to counter the fear of the unconscious. The analytic function of scrutinizing behavior, of consciously thinking and observing before participating, reflects a radical mistrust of unconscious impulses and their accompanying blind actions—some would say with good reason. As one gains in self-knowledge, one increasingly becomes equipped with a foreknowledge that enables one to avoid unconscious patterns of maladaptive behavior.

Psychoanalysts typically recognize counterphobic dynamics in their more unconsciously physical forms—hence, the terms *acting out* and *flight into health*. Perhaps because psychoanalytic tradition since Freud has advocated the taming of the irrational by the rational, of valuing thought over action, it has cast a relatively oblivious eye on the psychopathology of precocious mental activity, the involuted self-consciousness of "thinking in." For Otto Rank, the inhibitions of self-consciousness are a hallmark of neurosis. In speaking of the self-conscious neurotic seeking a cure by psychoanalysis, Rank (1936) noted wryly, "The neurotic has long since been where psychoanalysis would like to take him" (p. 251).

Psychoanalytic technique is a formal, systematic example of precocious mental activity that has been passed down in psychoanalytic training institutes from one analytic generation to the next. Clinical technique itself is a planned application of a therapeutic technology that adheres to certain rules and principles. In this general formal sense, the analyst, equipped with his foreknowledge of technique, may enter an analytic session precociously, before the session makes its actual appearance. With his correct technical principles in hand as a protective buffer, he can counter the phobia of spontaneously encountering the unpredictable intimacy of being alone with a person in need.

It is important to bring such heretofore accepted principles of clinical practice into radical question. First and foremost, we must question our assumptions concerning the juxtaposition of thought and action, of the conscious and unconscious, of planning and spontaneity. For example, are various analytic interpretations and interventions really more therapeutic for patients if they have been thought about ahead of time rather than offered spontaneously? Are we not adding another inhibiting superego, one derived from the analyst's training, on top of the superego the analyst already acquired in the process of normal socialization? Winnicott (1960b) has pointedly noted that the patient will not let his false self defenses down until the analyst has first done the same. Donald Schon (1983) has suggested that we replace such technical rationality with an alternate way of being with a patient, one that he calls "reflection in action."

Although it is true that through these various preparatory guises a person can avert the self-destructive pitfalls of unconscious impulses, what is gained in preparedness is always lost in an openness and sensitization to experience. Many adults who leap ahead and grow up too quickly might echo the sentiments of one patient who said, "I don't seem to be able to relax and have fun." Or as another patient said, "I feel like I missed a big party." The giving up of spontaneity may be too high a price to pay for the security gained through mental vigilance. There may be only sharp pangs of regret to show for the sacrifice of a full-hearted passionate life to the altar of the precocious mind.

REFERENCES

Balint, M. (1968). *The Basic Fault*, New York: Brunner/Mazel, 1979.

Bergson, H. (1889). *Time and Free Will*. New York: Harper and Row, 1960.

Ferenczi, S. (1909). Introjection and transference. In *First Contributions to Psycho-Analysis*, pp. 35–93. New York: Brunner/Mazel, 1980.

Green, A. (1978). Potential space in psycho-analysis: the object in the setting. In *Between Reality and Fantasy*, ed. S. Grolnick and W. Muensterberger. New York: Basic Books.

Joffe, W., and Sandler, J. (1965). Notes on pain, depression and individuation. *Psychoanalytic Study of the Child* 20:394–424. New York: International Universities Press.

Khan, M. (1974). *The Privacy of the Self*. New York: International Universities Press.

Kris, E. (1956). The recovery of childhood memories in psychoanalysis. *Psychoanalytic Study of the Child* 11:54–88. New York: International Universities Press.

Loewald, H. (1971). Some considerations on repetition and repetition compulsion. In *Papers on Psychoanalysis*, pp. 87–101. New Haven: Yale University Press.

McDougall, J. (1985). *Theaters of the Mind*. New York: Basic Books.

Rank, O. (1936). *Will Therapy and Truth Reality*. New York: Knopf.

Romanyshyn, R. (1989). *Technology as Symptom and Dream*. New York: Routledge.

Schon, D. (1983). *The Reflective Practitioner*. New York: Basic Books.

Shabad, P. (1989). Vicissitudes of psychic loss of a physically present parent. In *The Problems of Loss and Mourning: Psychoanalytic Perspectives*, ed. D. Dietrich and P. Shabad, pp. 101–126. Madison, CT: International Universities Press.

Winnicott, D. W. (1949a). Mind and its relation to the psyche-soma. In *Through Paediatrics to Psycho-Analysis*. New York: Basic Books.

—— (1949b). Birth memories, birth trauma and anxiety. In *Through Paediatrics to Psycho-Analysis*. New York: Basic Books.

—— (1960a). The theory of the parent–infant relationship. In *The Maturational Processes and the Facilitating Environment*, pp. 37–55. New York: International Universities Press.

—— (1960b). Ego distortions in terms of true and false self. In *The Maturational Processes and the Facilitating Environment*, pp. 140–152. New York: International Universities Press.

—— (1967). The location of cultural experience. In *Playing and Reality*. London: Tavistock.

11

The Story of the Mind

Adam Phillips

We seem never to ask "Why do you know?" or
"How do you believe?"
                              —J. L. Austin, *Other Minds*

One of the most famous, indeed constitutive episodes in the story
of the (Western) mind is the story Descartes tells of himself, as a
character, sitting alone in a room and practicing what he calls "extensive doubt." In his solitary quest for certainty—for that which
he can reliably depend upon to be true, to be really there—"the mind
uses its own freedom and supposes the non-existence of all the things
about whose existence it can have even the slightest doubt; and in
so doing the mind notices that it is impossible that it should not
itself exist during this time" (Descartes 1986, p. 9). This project of
ruthless doubt, this pursuit of the real, "frees us from all our pre-
conceived opinions . . . providing the easiest route by which the
mind may be led away from the senses." We are led, Descartes writes,
"to recognise that the natures of the mind and body are not only
different, but in some way opposite" (p. 10). Opposite meaning here,
in opposition to each other; but also, perhaps, suggesting that the
body and the mind may be mutual saboteurs. It is not exactly,
Descartes implies, that we need to get away from the body, but that
once we go in search of trustworthy foundations, of states of conviction, the body is the first casualty.

As we shall see, the mind object is that figure in the internal world that has to believe—and go on proving, usually by seeking accomplices—that there is no such thing as a body with needs. The body is misleading because it leads one into relationship, and so toward the perils and ecstasies of dependence and surrender (Ghent 1990); it reminds us, that is to say, of the existence of other people. In this sense the mind object is a perverse theorist of the body.

Descartes was not the first person to think of the body as an object of suspicion, as the enemy of truth. Finding ways of not being bodies, the quest for something better, for an alternative to the body— its desires and its death—is integral to both Platonism and Christianity. Truth or redemption is what we are left with once we are free of the body (as though it is the sin or error of the body that it is finite and therefore needs to be transcended). The need of the body and the death of the body make us think. For Winnicott, as we shall also see, it is a death, but a death at the beginning—a temporary psychic death—that prompts the locating of an extreme version of what he calls a mind. If, in early development, our "bodily aliveness," our "going-on-being," in Winnicott's words, is ruptured, if our existence is put under threat by an unmanageable environmental demand, we use our minds to maintain ourselves. Where there is a mind object at work there is a loss, or a violation, that cannot be acknowledged.

Descartes makes it very clear, although in a context of philosophical inquiry, that his very existence, his *belief* in his existence is under threat once he begins to doubt. Until, that is, he finds the thinking "I." "Descartes establishes to his satisfaction," Stanley Cavell (1988) writes, "that I exist only while, or IF AND ONLY IF, I think. It is this, it seems, which leads him to claim that the mind always thinks" (p. 108). For Descartes, thinking becomes the way people guarantee their existence (to themselves), establish their own presence in the world. My thoughts are inseparable from my sense of myself; indeed, they *are* my sense of myself, the only medium in which this sense can be. Like my home, they are where I live. For Descartes (1641), in *Meditations*, thought is the revelation that grounds him; his mind breaks his fall. "At last," he writes in the second meditation,

I have discovered it—thought; this alone is inseparable from me. I am, I exist—that is certain. But for how long? For as long as I am thinking. For it could be that were I totally to cease from thinking, I should totally cease to exist. At present I am not admitting anything except what is necessarily true. I am, then, in the strict sense, only a thing that thinks; that is, I am a mind, or intelligence, or intellect, or reason—words whose meaning I have been ignorant of until now. But for all that I am a thing which is real and which truly exists. But what kind of thing? As I have just said—a thinking thing. [p. 18]

From a psychoanalytic point of view—and in the context of this book on the mind object—Descartes's discovery can be, as it were, rediscovered. Is this not, for example, a precise formulation of some of the essential questions of childhood? What is inseparable from me, what is it I cannot bear to be separated from? And then, or therefore, what kind of thing am I? (and what kind of thing I am, or can be, depends upon that constitutive question of childhood, the litany of "how long?"). Faced with these fundamental questions Descartes comes to rest in his mind, or rather, as a mind, a thinking thing. Mind, intelligence, intellect, reason—words born of necessity, ensuring a future. As long as he thinks, he knows he is there, he knows where he is. But it is as though the mind is the only place left that he can be sure of being. One way of describing what he has discovered is that he is, in the telling phrase of Corrigan and Gordon, sufficient unto his mind.

From a psychoanalytic point of view Descartes's meditations may seem uncanny, germane even. There are clearly overlapping preoccupations but there is also the instructive jarring (of vocabulary and allusion; I am using, for example, an English translation of Descartes's Latin text) that should remind us that we are in different worlds. If a straight line cannot be drawn from Descartes's meditations to the psychoanalytic concept of the mind object—and it cannot, because to do so would be to omit such an array of contexts —useful links can nevertheless be made (Descartes's use of the paradigm of dreaming and waking is something of a lure). There is, of course, no place in the Cartesian system for the unconscious; but how does one make a place for the unconscious? If, as Gerald Bruns (1982) has written, Descartes "inaugurates a new era of epistemological thinking, wherein everything is thought to be determined or made intelligible by the workings of the mind" (p. 63), how is this different from Freud's psychoanalysis, or indeed, from Corrigan and Gordon's concept of the mind object? What stops psychoanalytic theory (and practice) from becoming a mind object? How can you make a system, a psychic apparatus, that includes what cannot be known? Despite the existence of the unconscious, psychoanalysis always tends toward a covert Cartesianism. How can psychoanalysis keep the unknown in the picture? How can there be a theory of the unknown, a knowledge of the unknown, as psychoanalysis sometimes claims to be?

I read Winnicott's extraordinary paper, "Mind and Its Relation to the Psyche-Soma," as a critique—a pathologization—of Descartes's meditations (it is characteristically Winnicottian in being a critique that makes no explicit reference to its object), and as a suspicion about psychoanalysis itself.

> *There is no meaning to the term* intellectual health.
> —D. W. Winnicott, *Human Nature*

Winnicott begins his paper with a quotation from Ernest Jones that he has found quoted by Clifford Scott in his paper "The Body Scheme in Psychotherapy." "I venture to predict," Jones (1946) writes, "that . . . the antithesis which has baffled all the philosophers will be found to be based on an illusion. In other words, *I do not think that the mind really exists as an entity*—possibly a startling thing for a psychologist to say" (pp. 11–12) (Winnicott's emphasis). With this assertion, which Winnicott will go on to confirm, he uses Jones to refer indirectly to Descartes, among others ("all the philosophers . . ." seems rather blithe). If Winnicott had read the sentence—and he may have—before the one quoted by Scott he would have found Jones in search, like Descartes, of foundations: describing psychoanalysis as a kind of Cartesian quest for essentials. "To ascertain what exactly make up the irreducible mental elements, particularly those of a dynamic nature, constitutes, in my opinion one of our most fascinating final aims" (Jones 1946, pp. 11–12). (When Winnicott refers in this paper to thinking becoming *a thing in itself*—an allusion to Kant's noumenon, that which the mind cannot by definition apprehend or know—he is, perhaps, cracking a philosophical joke. It is certainly the only explicit concession in the paper to what Jones calls "all the philosophers.") Where Descartes put the mind at the beginning of the story, Jones and Winnicott will put the body. But what kind of body? Replacing one term with another—dispelling the dualism of mind and body in the search for an origin, a true beginning—runs the risk of merely replacing one essentialism with another. The "truth" of the body may be just another way of getting us to believe in the Truth.

Endorsing Jones's assertion with one of his own—in the body scheme "there is no obvious place for the mind"—Winnicott (1975) draws a distinction:

> We are quite used to seeing the two words *mental* and *physical* opposed and would not quarrel with their being opposed in daily conversation. It is quite another matter, however, if the concepts are opposed in scientific discussion. [p. 244]

Perhaps it is paradoxical, at the outset, that the mind is to be replaced by the body, but daily conversation is to be replaced by scientific discussion in the search for truth. From a scientific point of view, Winnicott writes, there is "the development of the individual from the very beginning of psycho-somatic existence" (p. 243); there is a body composed of a psyche and a soma. We have to imagine the soma as the flesh-and-blood organism, a biological entity, and the psyche as "the imaginative elaboration of somatic parts, feelings, and functions" (p. 244) (it is not incidental, I think, that Winnicott does not define the word *soma*). If early development has been "satisfactory" the "mind does not exist as an entity in the individual's scheme of things." It is, Winnicott writes, "a false entity and a false localisation" (p. 244). The notion of a "false entity," of course, begs a lot of questions. The good mind, Winnicott will go on to say, is the part of the self that will develop an understanding of its environmental deficits, in the service of a self-reliance that can sustain contact with, and need for, the mother.

The bad mind—the "false entity" that Corrigan and Gordon call the mind object—reactive to the trauma of environmental impingement, tries to abolish both the need and the object. With good-enough maternal care, in Winnicott's particular sense of these terms, the mind would be, as it were, an ordinary participant in one's psychic life rather than an excessive preoccupation, a continuation of the mother one can take for granted rather than a substitute that one is continually rigging up. So Descartes's finding of himself as a "thing that thinks" becomes, from Winnicott's point of view, symptomatic—a description of a developmental deficit. The mind, far from being a virtual definition—indeed a location of—the essentially human becomes itself a distortion in the individual's psychosomatic development. What is at stake here, despite the special language—the albeit very different scientific discussion—of Descartes and Winnicott, is what, at his or her best, we believe a person to be.

Descartes's narrator writes of himself as "a thing which is real and truly exists" only as "a thinking thing." Winnicott (1988) describes children who have had to exploit their minds for psychic survival, and the consequent "unrealness of everything to an individual who has developed in such a way" (p. 140). In Winnicott's anti-Cartesian meditations, what he calls the mind is an attempted self-cure for a too-problematic dependence. Descartes depends on his mind to feel real. He is the "I" that thinks. Descartes's solution is Winnicott's problem.

It is misleading, as I have said, to assume a continuity of vocabulary here; words like *real, unreal, true, false, thinking*, and *I* are born of histories and contexts (and translations). But it may also be revealing to read Winnicott as wondering in "Mind and Its Relation to the Psyche-Soma" what might have happened to someone—a contemporary—to make him ask the kinds of questions Descartes asks in his meditations? What could lead you, at its most extreme, to doubt your own reality, to describe yourself, as Winnicott found some of his patients doing, as not feeling real? And how could one's

very existence get bound up with what one knew (or remembered)?
What is one relieved of, what is one managing, by certainty? Why
does doubting start, and what is its terror? Winnicott (1964) refers
in an early paper to "the child's most sacred attribute: doubts about
self" (p. 204). And for each person what kind of thing is a mind
assumed to be, and what kind of relationship can we have with it?
Indeed, where do we get the idea of a mind as something—an object—with which we can have a relationship (lose it, feel mindless,
say "never mind," and so on)?

In Winnicott's view, the mind is that part of the self invented to
cover for, to manage, any felt unreliability in the caregiving environment. It is, as it were, a necessary fiction, born of expedience,
and therefore potentially tainted by (unconscious) resentment.
Whenever the world is not good enough one has a mind instead.
"Here," Winnicott (1964) writes, echoing Descartes's opposition of
mind and body,

> in the overgrowth of the mental function reactive to erratic mother-
> ing, we see that there can develop an opposition between the mind
> and the psyche-soma, since in reaction to this abnormal environmen-
> tal state the thinking of the individual begins to take over and organise
> the caring for the psyche-soma, whereas in health it is the function
> of the environment to do this. In health the mind does not usurp
> the environment's function, but makes possible an understanding
> and eventually a making use of its relative failure. [p. 246]

In the absence of a relatively reliable environmental provision
the mind becomes a kind of enraged bureaucrat. Winnicott describes
the mind as "cataloguing," exactly and completely, unmanageable—
or rather, unimaginable—emotional experiences (in this sense the
mind object is the anti-type of the unconscious with its dream work
and its disregard for chronology). In states of privation thinking
"takes over," "organizes," "usurps." It is not incidental that Winnicott's language hints at political insurrection. He is, after all, describing an internal psychic revolution. In "health," one might say
using Winnicott's medical language, the mind listens to and collaborates with the body and its objects (or rather, subjects). In "illness"

there is a military coup and a dictator is installed called a mind object, at once bureaucrat and terrorist. The mind knows that it does not know, and it can use objects to find what it lacks; the mind object cannot bear the kind of knowledge called not-knowing. The mind thrives on ignorance; the mind object lives by convictions (and information). From the point of view of the mind object, at its most extreme, there can be no unconscious, because everything has already been accounted for. "A system," as Gerald Bruns (1982) writes in relation to Descartes, "is almost by definition that which contains no secrets, because it allows nothing to be set apart" (p. 74). But in a dictatorship, everyone is under suspicion. As Corrigan and Gordon (Chapter 1) write: "Patients who rely on their mind as an object, on some level, actually know all too well of its unreliability." A baby cannot bring itself up.

What Winnicott, and Corrigan and Gordon after him, alert us to with the concept of the mind object is the link between resourcelessness and the need to know. The mind, in Winnicott's account, is always making up for something, but something—sufficient maternal care—for which there is no substitute (any experience you need to know about, to understand, is a trauma). Knowing is the opposite of the false self-cure for dependence. "Acceptance of not knowing," Winnicott writes, "produces tremendous relief" (1949, p. 137). In Bion's complementary language one could say the mind object attacks the link between the person and his desire, and the desire and its object. So Winnicott's concept of the mind confronts us with a paradox that has significant consequences for the practice of psychoanalysis: *we only need to know, be mindful of, that which we cannot trust depending on.*

The mind simulates reliability; knowing is a cure for the erratic (or the contingent). What, then, of the kind of knowing that goes on in, is prompted by, psychoanalysis?

All those attempts to bring everything in around you are part of a naive belief that you can recreate the whole world. Well, you can't. Where would you put it? Next to the whole world?
                                        —David Hockney, *On Photography*

When Winnicott refers to "the overgrowth of the mental function reactive to erratic mothering," he gives us at least one description of the genesis of the mind object. *Erratic*, though, is an interesting word. The *Shorter Oxford English Dictionary* (1959, p. 630)
offers: "1. Wandering; first used of the planets, and of certain dis-
eases . . . 2. Vagrant, nomadic . . . 3. Having no fixed course . . .
4. Eccentric, irregular." Even though clinically we know what
Winnicott means by erratic mothering, after Freud we might think
of *erratic* as another word for the human; or to put it another way,
is the unconscious an erratic mother? Certainly all the words in the
dictionary definition would apply to Freud's description of the
unconscious. In other words, perhaps Winnicott in "Mind and Its
Relation to the Psyche-Soma" is writing not only of an interpsychic
experience—between mother and child—but also about psychoanalysis itself. Is Winnicott's "mind," for example, an unconscious parody,
or caricature of Freud's concept of the ego? And so is his paper a
critique not only of erratic mothering but of psychoanalysis as a
treatment in which the analyst strengthens the patient's mind? Or,
to put it the other way around, is mother also one of Winnicott's
words for the unconscious? If, at best, a person should, as Winnicott
says, "live as a psyche-soma," what kind of relationship, so to speak,
would a person have with his unconscious? What would a person's
life be like if he lived as a psyche-soma, relatively mindlessly? Would
the aim of a psychoanalysis be to know who you are, or to tolerate
and enjoy the impossibility of such knowing? Winnicott's paper, I
think, invites us to ask these kinds of questions.

Developmentally, Winnicott suggests, there was a time before the
mind, when there was nothing to know about and no need to know.
Once there is the trauma of impingement, once, as at birth, the
environment becomes excessively demanding, the mind appears. But,
as Winnicott implies, the mind is trying to know something that is
not subject to knowing (like, as it were, trying to look at something
with one's mouth). The paradox here—and this has difficult consequences for the notion of regression—is that the mental activity of
the mind object reinforces, secures, in a sense, the trauma it was
trying to relieve; the mind that takes over, sustains, by its very ac-

tivity, the discontinuity of being that is the trauma. *The mind turns up when it is already too late.* If the environment had been as it should have been, the mind object would have been unnecessary; its very existence signifies insult and betrayal (this is the root of hatred of the mind, of its very existence; for some children and adolescents failing at school is the only alternative to psychosomatic illness as a self-cure).

In the light of Winnicott's developmental picture it would make sense that in psychoanalysis one might aim to reconstruct the cumulative trauma that made the mind object necessary as a solution, but also to enable the patient to have access to that time before the mind. Does psychoanalysis, therefore, sponsor a more benign mind object—one, for example, that is capable of using insight about the genesis of its mind object—or aim to facilitate its absence, or both? Is psychoanalysis a way of teaching people how to get lost again (in thought)? Winnicott's concept of the mind raises the constitutive psychoanalytic question of the relationship between regression—even the ordinary regression of free association—and so-called insight. Where, if anywhere, in Winnicottian analysis does the mind come in? To which Winnicott's paper seems to reply, the mind always comes in afterward (to repair, to reflect, to reconstruct, to formulate, to consider, to fetishize, and so on). It is as though the project of the mind is essentially damage limitation. Why is it so difficult to imagine an analysis that consists exclusively of free association?

But because the mind always comes in afterward—after the trauma, after the state of absorption or free association—it always runs the risk of being a preemptive presence. The mind object, that is to say, has always unconsciously identified with the traumatic agent (or rather, events) that first prompted its existence; its function then becomes to impinge, to interrupt, to punctuate. *The mind that attempted to repair—to compensate for—the trauma becomes the trauma itself.* The mind, in other words, becomes the patient's cumulative—in fact, accumulating—trauma. A trauma that the analyst might feel some solidarity with.

My intellect, or whatever one usually works with, is also on vacation.
—Freud to Ferenczi, August 4, 1911

It was Ferenczi who first suggested that the patient is not cured by free-associating; he is cured *when he can free-associate*. It was, I think, Ferenczi's sense that psychoanalysis was potentially a form of mind object—a facilitating of the mind object, as it were—that in part led him toward his particular kind of courageous clinical experiments. His formative paper, "Confusion of Tongues Between the Adults and the Child" (1933)—an unacknowledged precursor of Winnicott's paper—is about the kind of trauma that makes a child knowing (and the kind of trauma that turns someone into a psychoanalyst). Psychoanalysis as a quest for reliable knowledge about the self (and the object) is a covert continuation of the Cartesian project; psychoanalysis as the facilitation of the (psychic) time before the mind—call it the capacity to free-associate, the capacity to be absorbed—is a very different project.

Psychoanalysis was born, in a sense, of the relationship inside Freud, between the Cartesian and the anti-Cartesian, the psychoanalyst and the dreamer. Both Ferenczi and Winnicott were struggling, I think, with the Cartesian in Freud and in psychoanalysis itself, what Bruns (1982) calls "the Cartesian collapse of being into the logically possible" (p. 80). And the logically possible becomes that which can be known. A psychoanalysis committed to the "logically possible" only seems like a contradiction in terms. In different ways Winnicott and Ferenczi confronted this irony by proposing experience—a certain kind of emotional experience—as an alternative to insight (or self-knowledge) as the legitimate aim of psychoanalysis. It is not incidental that Ferenczi, and his student Balint, and Winnicott and his students Khan and Milner, were pioneers of the idea of regression in psychoanalytic treatment. The word *regression* is a way of referring to those states of mind (or mindlessness)—either inarticulate or on the verge of representation—that defy or confound the already known. A regression is a revision, what Winnicott calls a surprise. The opposite of regression is not progress but omniscience. It entails the risk of entrusting oneself, something we do every day, without thinking, when we are momentarily lost in thought. Or in the kind of psychoanalysis in which we can forget ourselves. The idea of knowing oneself makes a fetish out of memory.

In the absence of trauma, Winnicott implies—as if there could be such a thing—there is nothing worth knowing. The concept of the mind object reminds us that we know things at our own cost, and that knowing is not the only thing we can do. Psychoanalysis can add to the story of the mind, the story of the mind on vacation.

REFERENCES

Burns, G. (1982). *Inventions: Writing, Textuality and Understanding in Literary History*. New Haven: Yale University Press.

Cavell, S. (1988). *In Quest of the Ordinary: Lines of Skepticism and Romanticism*. Chicago: University of Chicago Press.

Descartes. (1986). *Meditations on First Philosophy*. Translated by John Cottingham. Cambridge: Cambridge University Press.

Ferenczi, S. (1963). *Final Contributions: The Problems and Methods of Psychoanalysis*. London: Hogarth.

Ghent, E. (1990). Masochism, submission, surrender. *Contemporary Psychoanalysis* 26(1): 108–136.

Jones, E. (1946). A valedictory address. *International Journal of Psycho-Analysis* 27.

Winnicott, D. W. (1949). Mind and its relation to the psyche-soma. In *Through Paediatrics to Psycho-Analysis*. London: Hogarth, 1975.

—— (1964). On influencing and being influenced. In *Winnicott: The Child, the Family, and the Outside World*. Harmondsworth, England: Basic Books.

—— (1988). *Human Nature*. London: Free Association.

INDEX